Alone in a Crowd captures Andrea's eating disorder in a honest and authentic style. This ingenuous reflection of struggles and successes is sure to inspire and instill hope. We feel honoured that BridgePoint was able to play a pivotal role in Andrea's personal discovery and recovery journey by providing a holistic approach to eating disorders.

(Carla Chabot - Executive Director BridgePoint Center for Eating Disorders)

A tale of courage and honesty. It took many years and many struggles before Andrea was able to say "I'm Okay". It is a story that will positively influence others more than she even realizes.

(Dr. Herman Lombard - Psychiatrist FRCPC)

Alone

in a Crowd

A STORY OF A REGISTERED PSYCHIATRIC NURSE'S
STRUGGLES WITH BULIMIA AND MENTAL WELLNESS

Andrea Parmar

◆ FriesenPress

Suite 300 - 990 Fort St
Victoria, BC, V8V 3K2
Canada

www.friesenpress.com

Copyright © 2018 by Andrea Parmar
First Edition — 2018

Co-Author and Edited by Mick Parmar

Acknowledgements:
National Institute of Eating Disorders (NIED),
BridgePoint Center for Eating Disorders
Mental Health First Aid Canada
Eating in the Light of the Moon - Dr. Anita Johnston (Ph.D.)

ISBN
978-1-5255-2377-9 (Hardcover)
978-1-5255-2378-6 (Paperback)
978-1-5255-2379-3 (eBook)

1. *SELF-HELP, EATING DISORDERS & BODY IMAGE*

Distributed to the trade by The Ingram Book Company

I lift my head out of the toilet and hope it will flush. "Okay, all good. Thank God it did not overflow," I say to myself. I exit the ladies' washroom and head back to my booth at the restaurant. I chose this place because they have an "all-you-can- eat" buffet. I dish up my fourth plate of food and hope that the waitress doesn't notice how many trips I have made to the buffet table or to the washroom. Ten minutes later, I am back in the washroom stall to get rid of this bulge in my stomach. I'm pleased that I am all alone, as it definitely makes it easier when there is nobody around to hear me purge. It's time to leave, so I exit the restaurant, put on my lipstick in the car, and start driving down the street. I pull up to the Acute Psychiatric Unit and park my car. I walk in, and I'm greeted with smiling faces and the usual comments, "Hi Andrea, how are you today?"

"Great," I say, "I'm just fine." I grab a piece of paper from the desk and make my way down the hallway. It's shift change on the Psychiatric Unit, and I'm one of the nurses working the evening shift. I put on my happy face. I am ready to work and do what I do best … help people. I only have one concern. I hope that I don't faint because my blood sugar levels are so low after throwing up my entire lunch. I quickly slip a mint candy into my mouth and I am ready to go. Remarkably, I was able to live this lifestyle for sixteen years.

MY HOPES – YOU ARE NOT ALONE

Writing this book was not an easy decision for me. It was probably a troublesome thought for my husband too, as these pages would put my eating disorder, my deceit of family and friends, and our life "out there" for everyone to read and judge. However, now that I am in a healthier state of mind, I am able to not always "worry" about what others may think or say of me. At least not in the "people pleasing" way in which I used to obsess in the past. I realize that I never used to have the self-confidence, nor the tools, to think any differently. As a result, I was constantly searching for others' approval. "What they thought of me" was my foremost priority, with my own well-being on the shelf. With a life-changing shift in mindset, that took many years to accomplish, I have now learned to be there for my family and my close friends in a more meaningful manner, and even more importantly, I have learned how to take better care of myself.

You also should be aware that I wrote some of these pages over fourteen years ago, as the process began as simply a journal for reflection and healing. While you read my story, you may notice patterns develop and situations repeat themselves. The cyclical flow of this story reflects the very repetitive nature of mental health illnesses, addictions, eating disorders, and specifically in my case, bulimia nervosa. In my story, you will note many instances of despair, denial, and deceit. There were also plenty of moments of self-doubt, self-harm, self-awareness, and self-help. Much like a superhero movie, my life as a bulimic was an ongoing battle of good versus evil.

In addition, it is important to note that I was diagnosed with Multiple Sclerosis in February 2016. Currently, but I hope temporarily, I am unfit to work as a nurse due to physical issues such as muscle fatigue, balance concerns, and other dexterity issues. Obviously, nobody likes to find out they are ill, but I must say that this medical diagnosis has in some ways inspired me. It has motivated me to complete a journaling process that began many years ago and to also share my story publicly in hopes of helping someone. I guess it is my way of trying to make something positive transpire from the many years of self-harm. So thankfully, I have finally been able to find some peace with myself, including my MS diagnosis. I am determined that this medical issue will not become an excuse to give up on my hopes of trying to help others with their eating disorder struggles. Somehow, this new life hurdle has motivated me more than ever before to make a real difference in someone's life.

It is my hope that I am now mentally strong enough to be there for others with similar body image and mental health issues. I cannot discount the valuable guidance that medical and educational professionals are able to provide for their patients and our youth, yet I think I may be able to offer a different perspective. I have lived the life of a bulimic, and I have struggled with my own mental health. Somehow, I was able to navigate my way through that dark tunnel to a healthier lifestyle. So, perhaps I have a unique perspective. Not only am I a psychiatric nurse with some educational knowledge of eating disorders and mental health issues, but I also have the unenviable experience of having lived the life of a bulimic. I feel it is my duty, both as a medical professional and as a non-active bulimic to help others, so they too can realize a healthier lifestyle.

Did You Know?
Eating disorders have the highest rate of occurrence compared to ANY other mental illness disease. Eating disorders are twelve times more likely to lead to death than any other mental illness and thus are the most lethal and complex of all mental health disorders. (National Initiative for Eating Disorders)

I hope that you will in some way connect with the words I have written in this memoir, the life struggles that I have faced, and my tedious journey to learn how to love myself again. Addictions come in many forms; bulimia is just one addictive behaviour that I know a lot about since I lived it. The "cure" for every individual ... is just that ... a very personal, unique, and individual process. So your story is, without a doubt, very different than my story. That being said, no matter how individual our stories are, there are many similarities between bulimics and other addicts. Therefore, it is my wish that this book gives you hope if you struggle with an eating disorder, or with some other addiction. I will not pretend to offer you fail-proof solutions that will "cure you". I hope by sharing my story, it will reassure you that you are not alone in your search for a healthier lifestyle.

If instead, you are reading this book because you have a loved one who has an eating disorder or a mental wellness issue, then maybe you will be able to relate to my husband's thoughts included at the end of this memoir. I can admit, my eating disorder took a toll on our relationship ... our marriage was definitely put to the test. It may have bent, but I am very thankful that it did not break.

Did You Know?
Some mental health problems are more common than many physical health problems. While people often know a lot about physical illness, most people have little knowledge about mental illness. This lack of understanding promotes fear and stigma. It prevents people from seeking help early and seeking the most effective help. It also keeps people from providing appropriate support to friends, family members and people around them simply because they do not know how. In Canada, one person in three will experience a mental health problem in their lifetime. (Mental Health First Aid *Canada*).

In the end, no matter how dark some of your days may seem, I hope that you never give up on yourself, your partner, or each other. It will be a very difficult journey that requires much strength, patience, and reflection. I hope and pray that you, just like I did, are able to overcome the demons that haunt you and that control your being ... because contrary to what you may believe right now, your life is worth it, and many people truly do love you.

MY STORY

So here I go. True to my procrastinating past, I began journaling about my eating disorder struggles over a decade ago. This has been a long drawn-out process for me. I did not begin journaling with any thought of sharing my story with anyone, and I certainly did not imagine ever writing a memoir. It was simply a process I began and intended for reflection and healing purposes. Most of my life I have had a hard time "seeing things through to the end," and journaling was just another one of those things. Throughout my life, especially when I was sick with my eating disorder, my intention to complete new undertakings always seemed strong, but my motivation almost always fizzled. Similarly, I started journaling with much enthusiasm but lost my motivation several times over the years.

In retrospect, writing about my disorder played an important role in healing. However, I doubt that I realized the impact of self-awareness and the power of reflection at that time. Writing about yourself, especially your "deficiencies", is not an easy thing to do and probably another reason why I discontinued journaling many times. It was often very difficult for me to write *My Story* in an honest manner, as how does one write about your own dysfunctional life without telling any lies? How do you put yourself out there, for everyone to see, when it exposes a life that you are ashamed to be living? Or worse yet, especially due to my lack of self-confidence and fear of rejection, I wondered if anybody would even care to hear *My Story*. Once I slowly learned to truly accept and love myself despite my flaws, I was eventually able to overcome these concerns of humiliation and rejection … and I now realize this entire writing and publishing process is just another positive step forward for my mental health.

I gained the bulk of my confidence to truthfully write about my struggles with food once I was "bulimia free". Until then, there was plenty of denial about the seriousness of my illness. "Bulimia free" to me simply meant that I was no longer eating and then vomiting. It took three additional years of retraining myself before I could enjoy food in a healthy manner or without having to coach myself through consuming each meal. During these transitional years, my depression and anxiety grew, and I found myself needing a "new crutch to numb myself". Sometimes, but thankfully for a limited time, alcohol became my new drug of choice. Besides my husband, probably not many others would have ever guessed that I had some serious challenges. On the outside, I didn't look very sick and since I was still working regularly as a registered psychiatric nurse there were very few who knew about my struggles. During these difficult times though, I mostly stayed away from journaling. I now understand that it was probably the time when I would have benefited the most by getting my emotions out on paper, but that was a very difficult task for me.

I am evidence that journaling can be an effective healing tool. Many psychiatrists or other trained professionals who deal with mental illnesses will suggest writing your feelings down on paper. For years, as a psychiatric nurse, well before I began the process myself, I recommended journaling to many patients in my care. It's funny how we preach what we need to practice the most ourselves.

I am also proud that I have overcome a very harmful and complex behavioural addiction. One of my counsellors told me that bulimia and anorexia are ten times harder to overcome than other addictions such as alcoholism, illegal drugs, or cigarette smoking. If you think about that statistic, it makes complete sense. If someone has an addiction to alcohol, or even cocaine, part of the initial treatment plan would be to remove the substance being abused. Success would be based on the number of days a patient can go without using the substance. Unfortunately, this type of rehabilitation cannot be used for eating disorders. You can't remove food from a person's life to help cure them. We all need food to live. Ironically, I found out the hard way through my own dealings with body image concerns, it was actually the restriction of food that led me into a life of bulimia.

A NORMAL START OR SOME EARLY SIGNS?

"Your hair was so dark and thick," my mom said, "and you looked so cute in your pink sleeper." I was born on January 3, 1972 and had three siblings: two older sisters and one older brother. We were all born about thirteen months apart. We lived in a small three-bedroom bungalow in a close-knit neighbourhood of Regina. It was almost like a small town in ways, with kids playing together on the streets and in the playgrounds.

My dad was an accountant. He spent much of his time working out of town, so most days my mom had to take care of things at home by herself. She always made sure we were clean and well fed. Having four kids in five years by the time she was twenty-four is pretty amazing. I don't have any negative recollections from these first four years of my life as it seems like we had a very caring and loving home.

I also remember camping most summer weekends. Besides all the typical camping activities, that young kids loved, we used to also go from campsite to campsite asking people for their "empties" … as we were fundraising for a family trip to Disneyland. Dad would have the van idling on the road while my younger cousin and I would go in and "cutely" ask for the camper's beer and pop bottles. If we got the "go ahead", the SWAT team of older siblings would come rushing in and help grab every bottle we could find. Sometimes we hit the jackpot and other times we were told to scram … It was so much fun! Having three older siblings and several younger cousins was great. There was always someone to play with or get into trouble with. For the most part, it seemed like a very normal start to my childhood.

At five years old, it was finally time that I could attend school just like my siblings. I was probably one of the taller kids in Kindergarten, which is kind of funny because I'm currently 5'3". Like most people, certain events stick out in my memory of these early years. One of those memories is of a boy that I thought was cute, which sounds kind of crazy because I was only six years old. I was always trying to get his attention any way I could. At recess, my classmates and I would play tag. Actually, it was more like boys chase the girls. I wanted so badly for this boy to try and catch me. No matter how hard I tried to get his attention, he would always go after the other girls. I used to wonder why I wasn't good enough.

That year, in grade 1, my class put on a school play. My teacher chose me for one of the lead roles. I was to be the king and was really excited about it. I practiced my lines until I knew them inside out. My teacher told me that my character needed to use lots of expression. Being dramatic was easy for me, as I was not a shy kid by any means, so I was so excited to be one of the stars of the play.

Opening night was finally here, and I was feeling confident that I had perfected my character. The audience really enjoyed the performance, and everyone laughed at me. This made me feel great. I can still picture myself in my king's costume, with my grumpy personality like it was yesterday. I'll be honest, I really enjoyed the attention. I think most humans crave attention, but I not only craved it, I seemed to need it.

Like we see in the celebrity tabloids, there are many methods of getting attention. Some good, some not so good. Look at some of the famous people in Hollywood or those in the music or sports world. Usually, these talented artists and athletes are fan favorites because of their creative skillset or unique personality. To me, sharing these gifts and talents with fans is a positive way to gain attention. However, after a few years of living in the "spotlight" and dealing with the pressures of their lifestyle, some of these celebrities begin to make the news because of destructive or attention-seeking behaviors. Quite often, these dysfunctional public displays can be connected to an alcohol, drug, or mental health issues. Similarly, in my adolescent years, my need for attention and the pressure I put on myself to be accepted by others began to shape my thinking and spin my life down a path I never saw coming.

As we got older, many of my friends and I started playing ringette. My sisters, Tam and Kim, were already playing, so I was excited to finally be old enough to join them. The pre-school I attended was in a recreational centre, so I got the opportunity to get on skates by the age of four. I played for about eighteen years and have many fond memories. As the years progressed, the games got more competitive, and players needed to try out in order to make a team's roster. When I was around thirteen, I didn't make the travelling team, but my two best friends from school did. That bothered me. That year I played on a house-league team. We had a fun year, and I met some new friends. In one of our games during the season, we played the more competitive travelling team. Yes, the one that I didn't make. My dad said that he had never seen me play so hard before. We still got totally slaughtered, but I was okay with that because I was told by several people that I had a great game. My friend's dad even told us that he couldn't believe I didn't make the travelling team. I remember feeling good about that compliment.

The elementary school I attended was for Kindergarten to Grade 8 students. I liked St. Andrew. It was a Catholic school. My family was

Roman Catholic, and we attended church every Sunday. As kids, we all found it pretty boring. I understood the basics about Adam and Eve, Mary, Joseph, and baby Jesus. As a family, we all said our bedtime prayers as we knelt around our living room table. I can still recite that prayer in my head. Once we got to be teenagers, my parents didn't force us to attend church anymore, but strongly suggested that we should go. All of us, my siblings and I, pretty much stopped going except on special occasions like Christmas and Easter.

As mentioned earlier, I always looked forward to camping over the summer holidays. We would hit the parks almost every weekend. We usually went with my dad's brother, his wife and their two kids. It was only a forty-five minute drive to our favorite campground. We always had so much fun at Echo Beach, swimming in the lake, having camp-fires, and playing until dark at the playground. On a few occasions, when my cousin and I were just having fun, these older girls started calling us names and tried taking the swings away from us – for the most part, pretty common childhood bullying behaviour. My older sister, Kim, would always be the one to intervene on our behalf and put an end to the bullying. Thankfully, Kim has always had my back.

My parents occasionally went out on a couples' date night with their friends. As a result, we had several babysitters growing up. For the most part, they were great. We would have pillow fights and play other fun games. On one occasion, when I was about five years old, I remember getting tickled and wondering if the tickling was okay. All I can recall about the incident was that I really didn't like getting tickled in my pee-pee area … that tickling happened more than once.

I have some fond memories of my grandparents, however my mom's birth mom died at the age of twenty-nine when my mom was only eleven. Mom had three younger siblings. According to Mom, my grandfather did the best he could after such a loss, but my mom instinctively took on a mothering role. My grandpa got remarried when my mom was sixteen. We would always spend Christmas day over at my grandparents' house. All of the aunts, uncles, and cousins, about forty of us in total, would gather and always have a great time together.

My dad's mom, my other grandma, was also very special. She died when I was seven years old. I never met my grandpa on my dad's side as he died when my dad was only four and his mom never remarried. So it was just my dad, his two-year-old younger brother, and my grandma. Grammy would spend some nights at our house and often slept in my bed. It was a bunk bed, and my brother had the top bunk. Occasionally, I peed the bed. Actually quite often. I would wake Grammy up in the wee hours of the morning. "Grandma, I peed the bed. I'm sorry," I would say. We would both get up and change the sheets. You would think that she would tire of sleeping with me after a few accidents, but she didn't mind. She was very kind to all her grandchildren. I remember the day she passed away. She had a stroke. My dad and uncle had to break into her house because she wasn't answering the phone or the door. They found her on the floor. She died in the hospital about four days later. That was the first time I saw my dad cry. I still miss her.

So, like most people, I had many warm and loving childhood memories, along with an occasional sad one too. Heck, we even had a family dog. What more could I ask for ... Camping, family vacations, playing sports, a loving family, and great presents at Christmas and for birthdays. I wanted to be a kid forever.

THE DELICATE TEENAGE YEARS

By the time I was in Grade 8, I was one of the shortest people in my class. I was a healthy weight, but I really didn't think about my body. My friends were of all different sizes, and I was friends with just about anyone who wanted to be friends with me. Junior High years were thrilling. Boys, makeup, and school dances! I still recall the feeling I got in my stomach when I saw someone that I had a crush on. Despite that, I could hardly wait to get to high school because I saw all the fun that my three older siblings had partying with their friends. And before I knew it … I was there.

My oldest sister had just graduated, Kim was in Grade 12, my brother was in Grade 11, and I was in Grade 9. My siblings had definitely paved the way for me to have an active social life. I knew quite a few of the senior students, and I guess you could say that the Gilbert kids were fairly popular. I felt pretty proud on my first day, but admittedly, a little scared too. I think there were around sixteen hundred students in Miller High School, so plenty of new faces to get to know. I had a few close friends from elementary school that were in some of my classes, which helped with the transition. I even made some new friends in the first week. Before I knew it, it was time for the annual Frosh Dance. Every Grade 9 student got to vote for one girl and one boy to be named the frosh queen and king. On the morning of the dance, it was announced at school who the top three queen and king nominees were. Guess who was in the running? Me! I couldn't believe it. It was pretty flattering. Anyways, I was having fun at the dance with both old and new friends. Some of the older students asked, "Are you a little Gilbert?" Those questions were so flattering. Talk about feeling popular. I wore a pink skirt and a coloured top to the dance. Blue eye shadow, mascara, and blush made up my face. My hair, well let's just say it was big … This was the '80s of course!

The student council president came up to the microphone and announced that the frosh crowning was going to take place soon. Oh, how I wished I would win, seeing that my oldest sister Tammy had won when she was in Grade 9. A few minutes later, it was announced … "Your Miller High School Frosh Queen is … Andrea Gilbert!" My wish had come true. Talk about craving attention and the spotlight; I definitely had it that night. It had all the makings of a fairy-tale night for any teenage girl.

As the night was coming to an end, my long-time friend said she had something to tell me. First, she informed me that many of the girls that we knew didn't vote for me because they felt I already had too much going for me. I thought that was odd because I considered myself a friendly, modest person.

"Oh yeah," my friend continued, "Todd told me to tell you that he doesn't want to see you anymore." My stomach instantly felt sick, and I could feel my heart beating faster. Todd was a boy I had met over the summer and was my first high school crush. I couldn't comprehend how my night had turned so bad in a matter of minutes. A frosh queen one minute and rejected the next. I felt absolutely horrible. At the time, the night was simply a roller coaster of emotions, but now I realize that it was the beginning of bad things to come. It was a catalyst moment without a doubt that shifted my thinking ... I became an obsessive "people pleaser" because I never wanted to have my friends upset with me like that ever again.

With Frosh Week over, it was time to try and focus on academics. I had excellent marks in Grade 8, so I figured I would do fine in high school. It was a rude awakening as I soon discovered how much harder you had to work. My marks were definitely not as strong as before as my average dropped into the high-seventies range. I didn't worry about it too much though, because most of my attention was still focused on my social life. I continued to meet and hang out with new friends. This new group of friends mainly consisted of the "popular" girls and boys in the school. I weighed about 115 pounds then, but my weight was never really a concern yet. Two of my new girlfriends were absolutely beautiful, they wore really trendy clothes, and were quite slim. Even though I probably weighed about the same as them, I was still in awe of how they looked and the attention they got because of their appearance.

During our 1987 Christmas celebrations, my parents announced that they were going to take the family to Hawaii during the upcoming Easter break. This was a wonderful surprise. As Easter got closer,

I decided to lose a few pounds so I would look better in my bikini. About one week before our trip, I basically began to starve myself. I ate an apple or two a day and drank lots of water. One day, I went to the mall to buy some white Capri pants to wear on the plane. As I looked in the mirror in the store I got really shaky and became dizzy. I'm not sure if I really understood why I felt that way, or if I thought it wasn't that big of a deal, but I decided to add another apple and some orange juice to my daily diet the next day to take care of the problem.

Soon, the family was on the plane to Hawaii. The weather was gorgeous, the beach was breathtaking, plus there was delicious food everywhere we went. I was so hungry when we arrived because I didn't eat on the plane, even though I told my parents that I did. The next morning, we went down to the hotel lobby for breakfast. I will never forget the feeling that came over me when I saw all that delicious food at the buffet. I had lost about seven pounds in the week before we left, so I questioned myself, "Why can't I eat now? Of course I can, especially since I just lost a bunch of weight. Why should I have to deprive myself of all this delicious food when everyone else gets to eat whatever they want?"

I spent the next two weeks of our holiday eating what I wanted, when I wanted, and I forgot all about trying to look slim in my bathing suit. Our family had a great time lying on the beach and body surfing. I took a great suntan back to Regina with me. On my first morning back to school, I put on my white Capri pants and thought, "Gee, these pants are pretty tight. They sure weren't this tight three weeks ago." I wore them anyway. All my friends at school could not believe how dark my tan was and said, "Wow, Andrea you look great!"

Once again, I loved the attention I got, much like most teenage girls probably would in high school ... Well, maybe just a little bit more than most?

UNDERSTANDING BULIMIA NERVOSA

Here is a definition, some facts, and my own personal insight that may help you understand this form of disordered eating:

> **Bulimia Nervosa** – *"ravenous hunger". An eating disorder where one will binge eat and then get rid of the food afterward, by using laxatives or diuretics, or exercising excessively, or using self-induced vomiting.*

1. **Bulimia is an addictive tendency and a rollercoaster ride of emotions:** Bulimia was the primary "crutch" that I used to numb my body-image concerns, my negative self-concept, and my people-pleasing needs. Even though I was able to function "quite normally" at school, at work, and around friends, it was a very different story when I was alone. In order to gain control in my life and to fill the emotional voids, I would uncontrollably eat very high caloric foods. It is hard to explain, but I would get an "emotional high" with this sense of control over food … it was exhilarating. However, immediately after the binge, an overwhelming feeling of guilt would consume me. A panic-filled need to get the food out of my system just as quickly as I ate it, in order to not gain weight, took over. With the resulting purge though, a feeling of relief and calm would blanket me. These comforting feelings reinforced that bulimia was "my friend" and that it made sense in my life. The emotional tug-of-war battle, where I loved food one moment and hated it the next, was exhausting.

2. **Mental illness is the root of the problem:** Eating disorders are an expression of a mental illness. When it comes to my personal experience, I cannot truly say if depression and anxiety led me into a life of bulimia or if it was my body-image concerns and my

eating disorder that triggered my depression and anxiety. Quite similar to the "chicken or egg debate", I suppose it does not really matter which came first as both catalysts are probable. Either way, the evidence is clear, life-impeding guilt and shame are not only part of the bulimic cycle, but they are strongly connected to a mental health disorder.

3. **External factors can trigger Eating Disorders:** External factors can often put significant pressure on people, especially teens, by creating an image of what beautiful looks like. Whether it's on television, in a magazine, or on the internet, many dangerous and unhealthy messages are being relayed to our youth on a daily basis. I wasn't very concerned about my appearance until high school, but today kids are being exposed to these body-image "rules" at a much younger age … sadly, it's hard for kids to just be kids. The obsession to be thin, the need to wear brand-name clothes, the desire to be part of the cool crowd, or the pressure to become an elite athlete can all be catalysts for an eating disorder. In addition, being ridiculed or bullied by peers because of weight, body shape, or gender-sexual-diversity can also lead to depressive thoughts, negative self-worth, and a life of disordered eating.

4. **Bulimics are much harder to spot:** My average weight as a bulimic was around 115–120 pounds, at a height of 5'3", so what many would consider a reasonably healthy body-weight range. This very publicly-visible characteristic of this type of eating disorder is quite different than what you would observe in cases of anorexia. An anorexic's weight usually falls significantly below a normal or healthy range. As a result, their extreme weight loss and illness is easily detected by others. In my opinion, this lack of obvious clues is why bulimics are so much better at keeping their self-harming behaviour a secret from family and friends for many more years than those suffering from other disordered

eating illnesses (anorexia or overeating) or even drug and alcohol addictions.

5. **Bulimia can negatively impact your health in many ways:** I doubt the general population realizes how harmful and dangerous bulimia is to the human body. There are many organs and bodily functions that are affected by the stress of bulimia. I think it is important to bring some public awareness to the following list of medical consequences and risks:

- Tooth decay
- Low blood sugar rates
- Irregular heart rate
- Anemia
- Kidney failure
- Ulcers
- Decreased electrolyte levels and dehydration
- Esophageal ruptures (from excessive vomiting)
- Gastrointestinal problems
- Irregular periods
- Dry skin

I experienced at least seven out of eleven of these physical complications. Thank God I never tore my esophagus. Well, in one way I guess I was lucky, but in another way my "good fortune" just kept my bulimic cycle rolling along. The problem with my perspective at this time was that when a doctor told me that all my medical results came back fine, like when my barium swallow didn't show any tears, I was relieved. I wasn't relieved so much because I hadn't caused any permanent damage to my body yet, but instead my distorted thinking concluded that the doctor just gave me the "green light" to keep binging and purging … and that was music to my ears.

6. **Reproduction can be compromised:** My monthly periods were all over the place. After I got married, my husband and I were trying to get pregnant for about two years. With the severity of my disorder unknown to him, as I was still binging and purging during that time, it was truly a miracle that I ever got pregnant. Not only was I an "active" bulimic, but I also found out later that I had polycystic ovary syndrome, which also made conception more difficult. The following is a list of possible risks for an expecting mother who is bulimic:

- Miscarriage
- Stillbirth
- Gestational diabetes
- High blood pressure during pregnancy
- Breech baby (and subsequent C-section)
- Birth defects

A little later I will share more about my pregnancies and how much of a miracle both of my children really were.

7. **Counselling and medication support improvements to mental health:** Both counselling and antidepressant medication were beneficial to my mental health. Of course, you should always consult with your doctor to examine options in your recovery program.

8. **You will never "stop" being a bulimic or an addict:** Like most addicts, I don't think I will ever completely rid myself of the negative traits that led me to disordered eating. I would consider myself a "non-active" bulimic ... but now I know that the disorder does not define me. I think my body image concerns will always be present in one way or another, but I'm now okay in my skin *most* of the time.

In addition, according to the Mental Health First Aid *Canada* (2010) it is important to note that the *Risk Factors* causing eating disorders are complex and not well understood, and a combination of biological, psychological, and societal factors play a role:

Family History
- *Family members with an eating disorder (suggesting that there is a genetic component)*
- *Family members with mood-related disorders or who misuse substances (especially alcohol)*

Life experiences
- *Conflict in the home*
- *Parents with little contact with their children or high expectations of them*
- *Sexual abuse*
- *Family dieting*
- *Critical comments from family or others about eating, shape, or weight*
- *Pressure to be slim because of occupation or recreation (e.g. models, dancers, athletes)*

Personal characteristics
- *Low self-esteem*
- *Perfectionism (increases risk for anorexia, but sometimes bulimia)*
- *Anxiety*
- *Obesity (increases risk of bulimia)*
- *Early start of menstrual periods (increases risk of bulimia)*

I hope these defining facts along with my personal connection to bulimia nervosa will help parents, teachers, coaches, and others adults interacting with adolescents understand the scope and severity of this very dangerous illness. By raising awareness around the "Red Flags" or the "Look-For signs" of this mental illness, I hope that we can identify struggling adolescents well before it takes control of their lives. If we can identify early, then we can intervene at an earlier age and keep this ugly disease from ruining more and more young lives each year. ·

ANOTHER YEAR GONE BY

The school year ended with my final marks being in the mid-eighties, and I was satisfied with that. My weight was up a bit from the beginning of the school year, but nothing that I was too concerned about. The summer was here, so my friends and I spent a lot of time bike riding and hanging out in the park. It was fun, and I can't recall having any significant weight concerns then.

September 1987… I was in Grade 10 now. Wow, we were sophomores. My look had changed a bit. I wore a little more makeup and still had the big hair. My friends and I began experimenting with drinking, and I started smoking cigarettes on occasion. Ringette had started up for the winter, and I was now playing on the travelling team. Maybe not because I had actually made the team based on my tryout, but possibly just because they didn't have enough players. Nevertheless, I was happy that I was on the team. Numerous days were spent at the rink either playing or watching a sibling's game. One evening, while watching a game at the rink, a friend got up from the stands and went into the lobby. A few minutes later, I had to go to the bathroom. I got in the washroom and picked a stall. I heard someone throwing up in the stall next to me. I came out and headed for the sink and my friend was there. I asked her if she was sick. She replied, "Oh no, I just throw up sometimes when I eat too much." I thought that was kind of strange since I thought that people only threw up when they had the stomach flu or something similar. That was the end of the conversation, and we finished watching the game.

Did You Know?
The term "Eating Disorder" is unfortunate because it underplays the seriousness of it all. In fact, the "Disorders" are a serious brain disease with complex roots that manifest themselves through unhealthy eating behaviors. (National Initiative for Eating Disorders)

A few months later I found myself starting to obsess about how my clothes felt against my skin … particularly if they felt too tight. "Hey," I thought, "Why don't I just diet for a week, and then I'll lose enough weight to wear my favorite clothes again?" Little did I know that this decision to restrict my caloric intake would be another catalyst that led me into a life filled with disordered thinking and eating. Determinedly, I put my plan into action and I started to deprive myself of many foods. I was aware that I needed to eat enough in order to not pass out, but the plan was to eat the bare minimum. I began reading every single label on food containers, and I bought magazines about weight loss. "Lose ten pounds in one week … guaranteed," the magazines would read. I memorized the amount of calories in different foods: apple – eighty calories, banana – one hundred thirty calories, etc. My calorie-limiting diet plan lasted a couple weeks until a day when a group of us went to Burger King for lunch. My two "perfect friends" each ate a Whopper and fries. I ate a salad. This infuriated me. I thought, "How can those skinny, beautiful girls eat those burgers and fries and look the way they do? It's so unfair. I'm practically starving my ass off, and it's getting me nowhere!" It made me angry at myself and obsess even more about my weight.

For some reason, I cannot recall the first time that I ate and then threw up; however, I know I was around sixteen years old when the binging and purging began. My whole mindset started to change. Food became something totally different for me. I sort of had a love-hate relationship with it. I was always very careful not to get caught. If I was at home alone, I would check out the fridge, dish up my plate of whatever (it didn't matter), and sit on the floor in my room and shovel the food into my mouth. What a rush it was, until of course my stomach was so full I could hardly walk. I couldn't wait to purge this "stuff" out of my stomach. I never had to stick my finger down my throat. I just drank water from the running tap, bent over and out it would come. Some bulimics would have considered that a luxury, not having to use your fingers.

When I wanted to exercise my addiction at home, I had to get creative in order to not be heard. I would often tell my mom I was going to have a shower after I was done eating supper. As I share these memories now, my actions seem so gross. I can't believe the lengths I went to in order to hide my addiction. Sometimes, I would simply start the water in the tub and then throw up in the toilet while the water was running. I could flush the toilet several times with the sound of the shower drowning out the purging noises. Sometimes, however, I would throw up in the tub as well if the toilet was getting plugged. We were in an older house, and our toilet wasn't the greatest as it would overflow if it got too full. The first time it overflowed on me, I totally panicked. There I was in the bathroom with the shower running and puke coming out of the toilet. The floor was full of chunks of chicken, bread, and whatever else I had devoured that day. "Oh my God, what the hell am I going to do?" I thought. Luckily, I learned how to use a plunger in a hurry and got the toilet working again. The only problem now was the floor full of puke. I threw towels down and started cleaning it up. I rinsed the towels in the tub that was still running water. Now how long did all of this take and what the hell did my family think I was doing?

"What is taking you so long Ange?" someone would occasionally ask as they knocked on the door. "I won't be much longer," I would answer and pray that they would just go away. This addiction was very exhausting. Why would someone go through all this work? What need was it fulfilling? At the time, I don't think I thought about how hard it was to keep my secret. Or, if I did, I guess I figured it was all worth it. As time went on, it got harder to cover my tracks, so in turn I got more creative and more deceptive.

A GROWING ADDICTION

My mother was always baking, especially during the Christmas season. She would make dozens of cakes, cut them up, and stick them in the downstairs freezer. We were told that the baking was for Christmas, so please don't touch it. Well, guess what, I touched it. I would sneak into the basement laundry room, which was also our storage space, because that's where the freezer of goodies was hiding. Now of course, I had to wait for the right time to do this. What made things tougher was that my oldest sister, Tammy, now had a bedroom downstairs, which was right beside the freezer room. I definitely couldn't always wait for everyone to leave the house just so I could be alone. I was so damn sneaky. I would creep into the room, quietly open the freezer door, and stick my head in searching for the desserts. I can still picture myself holding a knife in one hand and delicately taking the Saran Wrap off the baking pan with the other. I got very good at working very quickly. Maybe it doesn't sound like it the way I'm describing it, but trust me, I worked fast.

The Hello Dolly slices tasted heavenly. Chocolate chips, condensed milk, sugar, and a crumb base ... yummy! Even though it was kind of hard to eat frozen, I did it. Then I would have to try and get the wrap back on the remaining cake. I thought for sure my mom was going to notice that there were some pieces missing, but hopefully not because there was so much baking in there ... anyways, the risk was definitely worth the reward for me. An added bonus to this basement was the new bathroom that my dad had recently built. It worked out great for my basement binges as I got away with sneaking goodies for a long time.

Occasionally my mother would think that she had more baking than what was in the freezer, but she never really grilled any of us kids about the missing goodies. Once Mom asked me about a chocolate square that she had put in the freezer. I told her that I had taken it to a friend's party. That was just one of the many lies I told. I feel so angry at myself right now. How could I lie to my mom that way? I have not completely forgiven myself for all the people I hurt with my lying. Maybe as I continue healing this will change and is probably part of the reason why I am sharing this story. Not only did my mom put hours of work into baking for our family gatherings, but she also made the best cabbage rolls ever. With my dad's help, she would take an entire day to make dozens of cabbage rolls. On occasion, I would help myself to a few. Unfortunately, at the time, they were so much more difficult to sneak and eat because they needed to be thawed out. At least I had enough sense to not eat a frozen cabbage roll.

By the beginning of Grade 11, my weight was about one hundred forty-five pounds. Even though I was throwing up my food, I still gained weight. I continued to be friends with just about everyone because that was really important to me. It still bothered me that some of my friends could eat whatever they wanted and continue to look perfect. As far as I know, none of my friends knew my secret. When a group of us were at a restaurant, I never ordered more than anyone else. When I finished my food, I would wait to see if anyone had to go to the bathroom. After everyone had gone, then I would go. If someone else was in there, I learned to be very silent. I didn't want anyone to know my secret. I say secret because that's what it was for me at the time. It wasn't a problem, it was just a secret.

As far as boyfriends went, I didn't have any. I didn't think I was ugly, but I know I thought I was fat. I wasn't sure why I was gaining weight because pretty much everything I ate came back out of my mouth. It pleased me that I was well liked by the group I hung out with. There were probably about twenty of us in this group, consisting of both boys and girls. We would party together on weekends. Like I said earlier, I was happy to be a part of this crowd because we were the "popular" kids in school … whatever that means. I also had some friends outside of this school-based peer group. My best childhood friend, Wendy, lived about five houses away from our home. She went to the neighboring public school. I spent many days at her house and we shared many sleepovers. Her mom and dad were like my second parents, and I am still good friends with Wendy today.

In 1989, I began my senior year. My weight was about one hundred fifty-five pounds. I always made sure that my hair was done perfectly, which meant teased so high that everyone would notice me. I soon found my friends coming to me for advice on problems they were having. I was a great listener and was always willing to help however I could. That was important to me and made me feel needed. Plus, then they would like me! And God forbid that someone didn't like me. Once again, the phrase "people pleaser" comes to mind. Well, let's face it, that's what I was. I was so worried about what other people thought of me that I didn't know how I felt about myself sometimes.

SWIM OR SINK

The faster I swim
The more tired I get
It's not a race
But I tend to forget

I want to get better
Perfection I crave
Everything is good
Until that big wave

I have to keep trying
I don't want to fail
I need to be seen
But not as frail

The tiredness continues
It takes its toll
My mood darkens
And I don't feel whole

Who am I trying
So hard to impress?
I know it's not me
There's others to address

I care so much
About what everyone thinks
But in the end
It's just me that sinks

GETTING OUT OF CONTROL

The binging and purging was now happening about ten times a day. One of my favorite things to do was to go out for a plate of nachos. I was still very careful when it came time to hit the bathroom. Since I was eating out more, my habit started to get quite expensive. So, I needed to get a job to pay for all the restaurant and junk food.

My first job was at a fast-food burger joint as a sixteen-year-old, Grade 10 student. What a perfect place for a bulimic to work. It was like heaven. As employees, we got fifty percent off our meals, so I would often show up early just so that I could eat before I started my shift. I didn't go crazy ordering too much food as people would for sure start asking questions then. Regardless of what I ate, it always ended up in the toilet. Like most fast food it usually tasted delicious, but it was full of fat and many empty calories. I only ate it for enjoyment of the flavors, but then it had to leave my body. It still amazes me how one minute I felt this totally "euphoric high" and then the next minute I would be filled with guilt, shame, and an overwhelming need to get it out of my body.

Did You Know?
Eating disorders are now the third most common chronic illness in adolescent girls. In Canada, 1.5 percent of young females, ages 15 to 24, report that they have an eating disorder. The average onset for eating disorders is 17. (Mental Health First Aid *Canada*)

I quit working at the fast-food burger restaurant after about one year because I was offered a new job at a yogurt dessert store. My assistant manager from the burger joint was going to be running a new franchise and asked me and a friend to come work for her. We both said yes. Wow, this was going to be awesome. I couldn't believe all the different toppings there were for the frozen yogurt. Chocolate bar pieces, cookie chunks, Smarties and mountains of other candy flavors. I had graduated from cheeseburgers to the desserts. Even better, I worked alone most of the time. Practising my habit was a bit tricky though, as the store was in a mall, and the washroom was down the hallway. That meant I had to leave the food court and quickly head to the bathroom to purge before a customer came up to the store counter. I worked quite a few Sundays, so there usually wasn't many people in the mall, which made it easier to disappear for about three minutes. I would get myself a big bowl of chocolate frozen yogurt and pile on the sweet toppings. I'd go into the back of the store and devour the entire bowl. A few times while I was stuffing my face a customer would ring the counter bell. I would quickly wipe my face making sure there was no chocolate on it and appear with a smile at the till. When this happened I had to be careful not to unintentionally throw up when I bent over to scoop up the toppings for a customer, since vomiting had become routine and almost a reflex reaction after a binge. I doubt that any customer or my boss would have considered that a very appealing dessert topping … thankfully, I never did.

LIFE AFTER HIGH SCHOOL

By the time I was in Grade 12 my grades had dropped to a seventy-two percent average. Luckily, I still managed to be accepted into Psychiatric Nursing, and I was excited about that opportunity. Just before graduation, a boy asked me to go out with him. David said he had liked me since Grade 9, so I figured he must really like me because I was a lot fatter by this time. We went to grad together and started dating regularly. My post-secondary studies started in the fall of 1990. I was taking nursing courses part-time and now working part-time at a drugstore. I was pretty overwhelmed with all the homework, but kept with it. I remember getting a bad flu just after classes had started in the fall. I didn't have much of an appetite, which was very weird for me. It was such a different feeling to not think of food. I must have really been sick. The flu lasted for about a week, and I noticed I felt a little lighter in my skin. I recall thinking to myself that even though I was no longer ill that maybe I should try to ignore minor signs of hunger in order to reduce how much I ate. It felt much like the first time I had started starving myself back in Grade 9.

Life continued on by attending classes during the day and working evenings at a drugstore. When I wasn't at work I was with my boyfriend Dave. We had officially become girlfriend and boyfriend. He had no clue that I was bulimic and occasionally starving myself. He did notice that I was losing weight however. Of course, like most boyfriends would be, he was impressed with the smaller version of the girl on his arm. I remember him trying to make decisions for me at restaurants at times. I'm not sure if he was trying to help me lose weight or if it was a control thing for him. I just know that he enjoyed having me by his side even more now that I was thin. He would say to his friends, "Doesn't Andrea look great?" It felt like he was showing me off to be honest. It seemed like he was saying, "Hey guys, look at what I got." I don't know for sure if this was the case, but that's how I felt ... like some kind of object or possession.

When we weren't around his friends, we did get along pretty good. He was a pretty funny guy, and he made me laugh. I remember the first time I met him back in Grade 9. He was a skinny kid with thick glasses. I had been friends with him all through high school. I always thought he was a nice guy, and I found him quite comical, but that's as far as it went. There was no physical attraction until the last year of high school when he started filling out and got contact lenses. Go figure. I had gone from frosh queen weighing in at one hundred fifteen pounds to this "porker" in less than four years, while Dave had gone from a skinny, "four-eye's" kid to a muscular, 6'2", pretty darn good-looking young man.

Even I was surprised at how fast the weight was coming off with my new diet. I probably ate about six hundred calories a day for a couple months. At work I was promoted from being a cashier to working in the cosmetics department ... I wasn't a beauty consultant officially, but I was really excited to get to know more about makeup and perfume. I was enjoying dressing up for work as there was a dress code in the beauty department. I got so preoccupied with my weight loss and looking good that I let my nursing classes suffer. I would get home from working until midnight and then try to study for an exam I had the next day. From September-November 1990, I had lost about thirty-five pounds. I was getting lots of comments from people, "Andrea, do you ever look good," or "Wow, Andrea have you lost weight?" I wasn't sure if I felt happy to hear the comments or disheartened. What did these friends think of me before? I can admit that I did like being at this new weight, however the pressure was now on to keep the weight off. I guess that's why to this day I don't like the word "diet". For many people the easy part is losing the weight. The hard part is when you stop following the diet. Most folks yo-yo back. They lose a bunch of weight in a short period of time, but when habits change the weight sneaks back on. Sometimes, they even end up weighing more than they did when they started the diet. This can be very hard on you emotionally, and that is why I no longer like diet plans.

It was about mid-December and classes were paused for the Christmas break. Out of the five classes I was taking, there were two that I was struggling with: human anatomy and drug therapy. Go figure. The other three classes were sociology, communication skills, and psychology. I had about an eighty percent average in those classes, which I was satisfied with. My attendance hadn't been very good though and human anatomy was definitely a class where attendance was important. There was so much content covered in the hour and a half class that it was sometimes overwhelming. What had I gotten myself into? Not that I felt like giving up necessarily, but the perfectionism in me was being put to the test. How was I going to handle all of the work ahead of me? It was not only school that made me feel like I was drowning, but my part-time job and my weight loss obsession added stress to the equation as well. My plate was full … no pun intended. I needed to succeed in all aspects of my life. I didn't want to fail at anything.

WAS CHRISTMAS REALLY THAT MERRY?

Christmas was going to be at my parents' house this year. My dad's side came over Christmas evening and my mom's side on Christmas day. My sister Tammy, her husband Darren, and my new nephew Jesse and niece Rebecca joined us. My sister Kim, her boyfriend, and my brother were there too. My boyfriend Dave and several family friends dropped in too. The house was always packed and many people complimented me on my weight. I was obviously thinner, and I didn't wear my hair so big. I'm not sure if there was a connection between the size of my hair and the size of my body, but both were proportionally smaller. Bulimia was still my secret, and I was good at keeping it that way. I enjoyed this time as our family was hilarious to be around. Usually my dad would have a few drinks and act silly with his Santa hat on. My uncle Gary would be his sidekick, but maybe not quite as tipsy. I knew there was going to be a loads of food and plenty of drinks, because that's what people do when they get together at Christmas, right? Since I was still dieting at this time, I wasn't sure what my plan for eating was going to be for the holidays. Honestly, I did fear that I would go right back to my old way of thinking … *All or Nothing*. I assume it is pretty common for people to overeat around Christmas and then get shamed into dieting afterwards by society and media ads.

As the people poured into the house, I got more and more compliments about my weight. At that time, I welcomed the compliments with a smile on my face. I could feel my self-esteem rising with every comment. Still, it was a bit scary, as I knew that the only way to keep getting the compliments was to continue to keep the weight off or lose even more weight. If I gained the weight back, I was not only fat, but I was a failure as well. Unfortunately, this was my distorted thinking and negative self-concept.

Traditionally, Christmas Eve was when we nibbled on appetizers as we didn't have the big turkey dinner until the twenty-fifth. Don't get me wrong, there was a huge assortment of food. Surprise spread, chicken wings, meatballs, spinach dip, and many other cheesy and deep-fried appetizers. Then came the desserts. Hello Dolly slices (minus a few pieces I had gotten into), cream puffs, butter tarts, and cookies. Despite having fun talking with everyone and having a few drinks, I really wanted to eat something. I figured that I should be able to handle a small plate of food. I dished up a small plate of the appetizers, and I sunk my mouth into the first bite of food. My mouth started to water, and a euphoric feeling came over me as I chewed the delicious food. The best way for me to describe that feeling was like an out of body experience where you feel like you are floating – like some kind of illicit drug that made you feel relaxed and excited all at the same time.

I ate everything on my plate and made a trip to the bathroom. I had a conversation with myself in the bathroom … mostly beating myself up for giving in. Talk about distorted thinking. I was doing the *all or nothing* again. I was definitely thinking "worst case scenario" during the twenty seconds it took me to get the "guilt" out of me. I felt so much relief once I finished purging. Of course everyone was too busy partying to notice anything out of the ordinary with me. After all, I was just eating and drinking like everyone else was. I even went to the bathroom for a pee like everyone else too. What was so suspicious about that? "Absolutely nothing," I told myself. So, I dished up another plate of the forbidden and fattening food. Because I was so good at being sneaky, no one ever saw that I was eating more than them. I would make sure that heads were turned the other way while I dished up. I would pretend to be watching everyone open up gifts, while picking up pieces of cake with a hand behind my back. I told myself that I deserved to treat myself tonight because I had worked so hard to lose weight. I wasn't going to gain the thirty-five pounds back in one night. I discretely gobbled treats down, while trying to be present in my surroundings.

Even when visiting with others, I was very cognisant of the timeframe between a binge and a purge. I knew that I only had about ten minutes before my body started absorbing some of the calories. As you can see, I was way too busy planning things in my head to truly be present and engaged with friends and family, especially during the holidays and other celebrations that were filled with food. Should I take another plate of cakes? Which bathroom was I going to use? How long could I wait before my body began digesting the calories? Was anyone keeping track of my intake? Did anyone hear me throwing up? If I threw up too much at one time, what would I do if the toilet overflowed?

Did You Know?
Bulimia nervosa is characterized by cycles of binging (compulsive eating of large amounts, usually sweet or high-calorie food) and compensatory behaviour (e.g. vomiting, using laxatives, excessive exercise). For this reason, the body weight of people with bulimia is normal or near normal. (Mental Health First Aid *Canada*)

My racing thoughts were interrupted when my sister told me it was my turn to open my presents. I put my plate of goodies down and found a spot to sit on the floor. I couldn't wait to finish opening up my gifts. The food I had just eaten was sitting in my stomach and making me feel guiltier and guiltier with each passing minute. I showed my excitement while ripping open gifts and saying my thanks. Now that my turn was over, it was time to get to a toilet and release all these terrible feelings. At the time, I only knew how I felt physically and emotionally. I wasn't even close to trying to analyse this illness from a cognitive or mental health perspective. Truthfully, at the time I didn't even think I was ill, so there wasn't anything to try and figure out. All I knew was that I didn't want anything left inside of me that could cause me to gain weight overnight. I had a few more drinks with everyone and helped my mom clean up and called it a day. Tomorrow, Christmas Day, was another big day.

Most people were looking forward to Christmas day, but not me. Like I mentioned before, I was scared that I would slip back into my old patterns. I was excited about the holiday season a few days ago, but since I had purged this evening, I wondered how I would manage tomorrow. I made a deal with myself. I would take a break from eating and then *not* throwing up. When the New Year was here, I promised that I would begin restricting my intake again. I had made a plan. It all sounded good to me. My head hit the pillow with a smile across my face. Now I was really looking forward to tomorrow. I would be able to treat myself and eat as much as I wanted. Of course, I would have to plan my binges and make sure no one was monitoring my intake. I would fool everyone.

When I woke up, the first thing I thought of was all the food that I was going to eat today … actually it was also the last thing I had thought about before falling asleep too. A buffet of turkey, cabbage rolls, mashed potatoes, gravy and all of those wonderful goodies that my mom had spent days making. To be honest, I didn't really care who made the food. Food was food. There was a tray of dainties on the counter from the night before. I immediately began figuring out how to get a few pieces of cake without my parents noticing. I mean really, who eats chocolate squares first thing in the morning? Me, I guess. When I was preparing for a binge that was all I thought about. I would go into some sort of trance. Almost like being hypnotized I imagine. That maybe sounds crazy, but that's what it was like for me. There wasn't anything normal about the thoughts that went through my head which kept me from being truly present in the moment. At my worst, I could be in a room full of people, yet I was very *alone*. I was not only disconnected from the people and the conversations in the room, but from my feelings as well. I was clearly addicted to my eating behaviors as I was consumed by thoughts of my next binge. I craved the rush I got from planning and executing the process. I floated along in the sky, nowhere near the ground.

I was able to snatch about four pieces of dainties quite easily. My parents were arguing over how to stuff the turkey properly, which was funny for a brief moment. I hurried to my room and was pretty much slobbering onto the carpet by the time I got there. I knew I had a glass of water in my room, which I needed to throw up properly and safely. Otherwise, the food would get stuck in my throat on the way out. It probably took me all of three minutes to devour the sweets. The rush had ended. Now it was time to get this stuff out of me. Since it was a smaller amount of food, I just threw up in my bedroom using the cup I drank the water from. This was something I did quite often. Then when I went to the bathroom, all I needed to do was dump the cupful of puke into the toilet and flush. That helped cut down on the time I was in the bathroom. It would seem like I had just gone in there for a quick pee ... an ingenious plan for sure.

By the time the rest of the family arrived for our Christmas Day supper, I had already had about four mini-binges. We all settled in at the dining room table and said grace. My dad added how happy he was that we were all together and wished us all good health. "Speed it up, Dad. Let's skip the prayers and well wishes, and start eating," I thought. I ate and ate and ate and barfed and barfed and barfed. I can't remember how many times, but it was a lot. I took smaller helpings so no one would say, "Oh Ange. Are you going to eat all that?" There was also plenty of conversation during the meal, but I can't remember much of what we talked about as I was consumed mostly by my own trains of thought.

When we have physical issues we go to the doctor and get something to relieve the pain. With emotional pain, it's a lot more difficult, and sometimes there is a stigma attached to that type of pain ... you're weak, you're unstable, and maybe even, you're crazy. It's getting better, but in the past, people were ashamed when anti-depressants and therapy sessions were prescribed. I often wondered why I chose to become a psychiatric nurse versus a regular nurse. I knew from a young age that I liked helping people with their problems. Usually the problems were trivial ones, but nonetheless, I was the one people went to. And if they didn't come to me, I went to them. I felt like it was my duty to make people happy. If everyone around me was happy, then so was I. If anyone was sad or mad, I would then assume that it was either my fault or it was my responsibility to make them feel better. I would try my best to put a smile on their face as I didn't want to feel bad either.

If I received the smallest amount of disapproval from one person, my whole mood was shattered. It never occurred to me that if someone was rude or mean that they might be dealing with their own issues. I admit, just like most of us, I have criticized or disagreed with some acquaintances in the past. As life would have it, we are not going to like everyone we meet nor is everyone going to like us. I would be surprised if my opinion has ever had the power to make others feel worthless. Yet, when someone disagreed with me or used a tone of voice that seemed unpleasant, I internalized that message in a self-defeating manner ... I took it very personally, when most likely it wasn't meant to come across that way. Without a doubt, because of my fragile self-worth and mental health, I was much too sensitive. I needed to learn that I was not worthless just because others did not agree with my opinion. I still occasionally struggle to maintain this "thicker skin", as reducing my need for other people's approval is still a work in progress. My resilience has improved, as I'm not as delicate as before, but I can also admit that the negative thoughts still creep in once and a while.

Back to Christmas day. After we finished our big dinner, we opened up a few more presents. My boyfriend had come over by that point. Another set of eyes to watch me. I can't even tell you how many calories I took in that day. I assume at least ten trips were made to the bathroom to purge. It was a vicious cycle, but I promised myself that I would stop this crazy behavior come the New Year. I would enjoy all the rich foods that the season brought and then come January 1, it would be time to make a change. I also knew I needed to pull up my socks in school, as I really did want to be a psychiatric nurse.

MAKING AND BREAKING PROMISES AGAIN

Happy New Year everyone. Although I am not certain what I did to bring in the New Year, I do remember breaking the promise I made to myself. Once again, I set myself up for failure. I was so proud of myself when I had decided that the New Year would be "bulimia free", but only to let myself down again.

THE CYCLE OF BULIMIA

The cycle begins
With the cravings I fight
I try to avoid them
With all of my might

I quickly surrender
To the desire within
I head for the food
And the binge begins

Of course this is a secret
No one knows but me
That's part of the cycle
That I really like to see

Being able to eat
Those forbidden foods
Gives me a high
In all of my moods

I finish indulging
The high comes to an end
I need to fix this
As I can hardly bend

It doesn't take long
To rid all the guilt
Then I'm back to normal
This is how I am built

It was around this age that more notable signs of depression began manifesting. I had self-esteem issues for quite some time, but I remember a definite change in my mood. I began having waves of varying emotions that I couldn't explain, and they were occurring much more frequently than ever before. Wherever the feelings came from, they made me cry. It's hard to remember everything clearly, especially when it comes to actual dates, as most days were just a blur to me. Nursing classes resumed and I continued working at the drugstore. I really needed to start focusing on those two classes that I was falling behind in, but luckily I was still doing well in the other three classes. I turned nineteen years old on January 3, 1991. I was pretty excited because I was now of legal drinking age and I could buy my own liquor.

Kim, Geoff and I still lived with Mom and Dad in the Douglas Park bungalow, but my parents were looking at getting a larger home. We had been in the same house for about twenty-one years. I was excited for them and eager to help out. They were looking for a home in University Park, which was about a five minute drive away from their current address. One day when I was home alone a couple shopping for a new home came by to view our house. Thankfully, I wasn't in the middle of a binge, so I was able to show them around. I really enjoyed playing real estate agent. They thanked me for the tour and called later that night with an offer that my parents accepted. My dad had said he would give one hundred dollars to whoever "sold" the house. I was pretty darn proud of myself.

My dad was out of town with work for the week so it was up to Mom and me to look for a new house. There were a few open houses in the area we wanted, so we headed out on our search. We found a two storey that was perfect. If we purchased it, I would have my own room. It had a sunken family room, two car garage and a fireplace. We loved it. My mom put in an offer, with the understanding that my dad had to view it as well. When my dad saw it the next day, he approved. We were now the proud owners of a new home. I guess it wasn't really my house, but that didn't stop my excitement. I recall that I was very aware that there were three toilets in the new home. I would have more selection and less chance of getting caught. Ironically enough, I would now be living just around the corner from my boyfriend. We got settled in our new house sometime in the spring. I loved my new bedroom, and I had already "christened" all of the toilets. They all flushed perfectly, which was another bonus for me. Things were looking up for me, or so I thought.

It was getting close to the end of the semester in school, and I was trying my best to be studious. The passing mark for our exams was eighty percent. We usually had two exams per week throughout the semester. If you failed an exam, you were allowed one rewrite. If you failed your rewrite, the instructor would examine how you were doing in your other classes. This had happened to me once in my human anatomy class. My instructor believed that I had the potential to be a nurse, and even complimented me on my easy-going personality. She recommended I retake the class next year. However, I would not be able to start the second year of studies until I completed this class. I was disappointed at first, but then thanked my lucky stars that I hadn't been dismissed out of the program entirely as some other students had been. I decided that I should redo my drug therapy class as well. I had passed it previously, but I felt that I should try to improve my mark. So that meant in the fall semester I would take just those two classes. My parents were disappointed at first, but were supportive of my decision to continue on in the program.

During this period, I was purging about five to ten times a day. If I ate something in front of other people, it wasn't very much. When I was by myself, I would escape into my own world and binge away. I had thought that once we moved, I would be able to alter my behavior. Who was I kidding? I was the one that was so excited about the multiple bathrooms and my new bigger bedroom. It had a huge closet too, which meant more room to store my binge food. I could eat what I wanted, when I wanted, and no one was there to tell me to stop. This was my preferred state: escaping reality, and getting a high from my addiction. There was just one problem. I think my parents were catching on to me. I honestly can't recall the exact day that they began suspecting their daughter had an eating disorder or other mental health issues. Maybe my mom can. I have never really asked her. Food items kept disappearing, so my parents started asking questions. "Geez, Mom. I don't know where that box of chocolates went." Or, "No Dad, I didn't eat that container of sliced meat." I'm ashamed of the lies that I told to the people I love.

Did You Know?
Binge eating is often done in secrecy; however, individuals may begin binge eating in a restaurant and continue upon returning home. Most people are ashamed and distressed by their loss of control over eating, which makes them easier to engage in treatment, although there is typically a delay of many years before they seek help. Bulimia nervosa usually begins in late adolescence, affecting mostly women. Between 1.1 and 4.2 percent of women will develop bulimia. The rate of occurrence in males is approximately one-tenth of that in females. (Mental Health First Aid *Canada*)

One day, my parents found some food wrappers in my room. I'm not even sure what kind of wrappers they were, I suppose that is irrelevant. When they confronted me, I admitted that I would sometimes sneak food, eat too much of it, feel sick to my stomach and then throw up. Even though I downplayed my issues, I could tell my parents had their suspicions that something wasn't quite right because they did not seem shocked at all. They told me that I was a special person and had many positive characteristics. They didn't care what my weight was, they just wanted me to be happy. I told them that I would stop throwing up. They, of course, didn't know how bad my addiction really was. They only knew what I had told them about my addiction, which was mostly lies. The worst part is that I felt empowered by this confrontation. I told them just enough to get them to feel sorry for me and get off my back so I could just continue what I enjoyed doing most. Without a doubt, I manipulated the situation to get what I wanted when it came to food. I would just have to be a bit more careful in covering my tracks in the future. I was ready for the new challenge.

FLOWER GIRL

Summer was finally here. This was my first summer since my "weight loss" and my newfound "ability" to not to gain all the weight back. I had recently bought some new shorts and tank tops, and I couldn't wait to show off my new and improved body. I was still working at the drugstore when I got another part-time job at a flower shop close to home. I just happened to go in there one day and asked the lady working if they were hiring. I got a call the next day from the flower shop owner. Dena offered me a position, so I accepted and submitted my resignation at the drugstore. The new job was great. It was in a small flower shop that was part of a chain of larger stores. Dena had a fridge full of beautiful flowers and stocked many beautiful plants. I always loved flowers, so I was looking forward to working there.

Dena trained me on the cash register and other opening and closing duties. I would be working by myself often as the two of us were going to job-share. The new position would work well with my upcoming fall class schedule. The days I was off school, I would work. My wage was slightly above minimum, so I earned enough to get by as my parents weren't charging me rent as long as I was enrolled in school. I didn't have a vehicle back then, but my mom and dad let me drive their van.

On my first afternoon at work, I watered all the plants and flower arrangements in the store. They were so gorgeous. Dena had the store arranged so nicely. It was a very welcoming little flower shop. She was a very particular businesswomen, and she wanted to keep the store looking that way. I liked that about her. The store was in a small strip mall, so it wasn't really busy. There was a drugstore and a pizza joint in the mall as well. The store had a front display room and a larger prep room in the back. We got flower deliveries twice a week from the main store. All of the fresh flowers needed to be cut and put in buckets. There were artificial flowers and other items stored in the back room too. And of course, most importantly, there was a staff bathroom. The toilet was old, but worked just fine. Always a selling feature in my eyes. Yes, I had the perfect job. I loved flowers, I enjoyed talking to new people, and I was able to walk to work. The day flew by, and it was soon closing time. I cashed out and filled out the deposit sheet. The store was organized and tidy. Everything went perfect on my first afternoon of working alone.

On my first Saturday of work, I was there by myself from opening to close. I was allowed one hour for a lunch break. The phrase "lunch break" didn't really mean a whole lot to me. To me, it simply meant that I was able to leave the store for up to one hour. The "lunch" part didn't really register, as I soon began eating and purging all day long at the flower shop. Don't get me wrong. I was still able to function and do my job well. To look at me, customers would have never guessed that I had an issue. I was always looking my best, and I was very friendly to everyone. I was a good employee despite my addiction. I even took the time to learn more about flowers as there was plenty of reading material in the store. As my boss encouraged, I experimented with fresh cuts and made some pretty arrangements in my spare time. I don't think, however, that Dena would have been very happy with me practicing my eating disorder at the flower shop. I had a "back in five minutes" sign that I would put on the door, which gave me just enough time to run across to the drugstore to buy bags of chips and a bunch of chocolate bars. I hid my bag of goodies in a cabinet in the back room. I sat down and started gobbling as soon as I had a free moment. There was a swinging door between the front of the shop and the back room. A bell also chimed when someone entered the store, which gave me plenty of warning. Even though I never got caught, sometimes a customer would come in while I was in the bathroom throwing up. I would just stop, flush the toilet and walk into the display room. "Good afternoon! Can I help you find anything today?" I would ask with a big smile on my face ... it was going to be a great summer.

SCHOOL, WORK AND BINGING ... ALL IS GOOD?

September 1991 – Here we go. Round two for these two classes. I was determined to improve my marks in both of them by being more studious this time around. I had no excuse for not doing well. I should be able to. Anyone else would, right? I once again tried having a new outlook on life. The plan was that right after the Labour Day long weekend I would stop binging and purging for good. I planned to spend my time focusing on my studies and getting into shape. I even got a membership at a fitness gym. Like every other time, I started the new plan with a determined effort. I was doing really well in my classes, and I was regularly attending an aerobics class at the gym. I was even able to go a full week without throwing up. After classes, I worked at the store until 6:00 p.m., and then I was at aerobics ten minutes later. Once I started purging again, I just made sure that I had some juice in my system. That kept me from passing out. Boy was I a genius.

The months went by and Christmas was approaching. I made some new friends at school, which was great because I wanted to be friends with everyone. I assume my parents had some suspicions that I was occasionally throwing up still, but I really doubt they had any idea how complex and serious my behaviors were becoming. I started buying my own "binge food" because I knew I couldn't continue eating their food, especially with my dad being "hawk eyes" when it came to food. Honestly, he would notice the smallest thing missing from the fridge. If there were six hamburgers left from supper, the next day he would come home from work and check the fridge. I think he counted them before he went to bed. And I know what you are thinking ... you spot it, you got it ... and you are right, I always had inventory of what was in the fridge too.

Of course my dad's behavior frustrated me. It made my life much more difficult. My mom, on the other hand, didn't notice as much when things went missing. Like the money from her wallet, or the bag of broken gold chains that she planned to get melted down and made into a ring. I knew the pawn shop downtown wouldn't give me what the gold was worth, but I didn't care. It was money and that meant food ... Sorry, Mom. I feel terrible about my past dishonesty. Everything that I did seemed to be centered on food. I guess that was not totally true as I was doing really well in school. My mark in human anatomy was around ninety percent while my drug therapy mark was in the low eighties. I was focused on my studies and was attending every class. I was happy that my efforts were paying off. When it came to being a student, I could feel a positive change in my attitude and my confidence. Now that I was attending class regularly and doing all my homework, I wanted to keep excelling.

I couldn't believe Christmas was almost here, again, but I noticed a difference in my level of anxiousness. Last Christmas, I was feeling very pressured because I had lost a bunch of weight prior, and I was struggling with the decision whether I should binge or not. This year, I didn't feel any pressure of making a choice ... I was at peace with the fact that I was going to binge and purge during the holiday season. My "new and improved" attitude regarding my eating disorder relieved some stress. I guess what I mean is that because this habit had now become a way of living for me I wasn't so anxious and guilt-ridden ... I just accepted that it was part of who I was. I was much more aware that I was bulimic. I knew what I was doing, and I was fine with it.

ADDICTION AWARENESS

Addiction I know
Comes in different forms
It's too much of something
Beyond the norms

Just stop the behavior
People would say
They don't understand
The attempts made each day

You have to be ready
But what does this mean
There will be no big signal
That appears on your screen

Awareness to the problem
Is step number one
But that's where we get stuck
Because we think we are done

Sometimes we hang on
Because it's our friend
What we don't understand is
It's the beginning of the end

So yes, I was now making a conscious decision to binge and purge. Maybe I wasn't fully aware of how unhealthy my lifestyle was yet, but I had acknowledged that it would just be a part of my life. Instead of beating myself up over it every day, this form of "eating" just became my norm. I seemed a bit more present when talking to family and friends, even while I was eating food, because I had a routine and that relieved a significant amount of stress for me. In an odd way, I figured that this was a healthier decision. Of course, in actuality it was the exact opposite of healthy. My eating disorder was now who I was and second nature to me.

JUST ROLLING ALONG

January 1, 1992 – Happy New Year everyone! Dave and I were at a house party. We had been dating for about a year and a half. He was a pretty good boyfriend, I guess. He bought me nice gifts. He still had no idea what I was doing with food. Like most bulimics, never getting caught was one of the biggest stressors of my disorder. I was a "closet" eater and very deceptive in my efforts to purge.

I was still working at the flower shop and learning more about products and making the arrangements. I continued to buy large amounts of junk food from the nearby drugstore. Again, it was who I became, and I didn't see anything wrong with what I was doing. By this point, I would estimate that I was consuming between five and seven thousand calories a day.

I am going to take a moment to share a passage from an inspiring book that I read about disordered eating by Anita Johnston (PhD) called *Eating in the Light of the Moon* (Gurze Books, 1996):

Many women do not recognize the addictive nature of disordered eating until they find themselves in the throes of it, mercilessly driven by a compulsion for thinness and hounded by an appetite for food that seems insatiable. They find themselves unable to silence one inner tyrant that hollers, "I want more, more, more!" while trying to appease another who rejects anything short of the perfect body as not good enough.

Wanting desperately to be free from this addiction, they despise their voracious hunger, and loathe their imperfect bodies. Because they misinterpret their hunger as physical, they see food as the enemy and their bodies as traitors in a war against fat. Caught up in the denial that is ever present in all addictions, they fail to recognize the starvation of their spirits. They cannot see the emptiness that is in their hearts. They make a fundamental error in failing to separate what is concrete from what is symbolic and become obsessed with the concrete object, the food itself. They do not see that the addictive object is a representation of something much greater, that it is only a symbol of what they truly desire. They do not understand that the terrible emptiness they feel is a spiritual or emotional emptiness, not a physical one.

Spring was here, and I felt like life was on the upswing. My marks had improved so much that I was asked to tutor fellow classmates. I could tell you the name of every bone in your body, the functions of organs, and the classifications of prescription drugs. I achieved a ninety-five percent in human anatomy and eight-five percent in drug therapy. After discussing my improved progress with the program's student counsellor I decided to continue with the part-time option, so that I could also continue working at the flower shop to pay for my schooling (and my addiction). As a result, I had two years remaining in order to complete my diploma.

Socially, Dave and I went out with friends on weekends and occasionally watched movies at each other's house during the week. He was still living with his parents too. The money I was making at the flower shop wasn't great, so I found the need for a little more cash flow. On a whim, I decided to stop at the government run liquor store in our area to see if they were hiring. A man greeted me when I walked in. He happened to be the manager. I gave him my resume and he told me that he would call if they needed any part-time help. About a week later, the manager called and offered me a casual position. I accepted immediately. At the time, minimum wage was $5.50/hr, so I knew it would be significantly better than that. This job would be great to have while I was in school too. I could work on weekends and during the holiday season.

John, the manager, had me come in a few days later for an orientation shift. I was introduced to Janice, who had been working there for several years, and she would mentor me. I spent most of the day learning how to operate the cash register. I had much to learn about the many products, but I was up for the challenge. Just before I was ready to go home for the day, John told me my starting wage would be $12.00/hr. Wow ... that would be great. I could work ten hours a week and it would be the equivalent of working about twenty-two hours a week at the flower shop. To be fair to Dena, I didn't want to quit the flower shop right away. I told her about my new job, but I knew that I wouldn't be able work Saturdays for her anymore as that was the main day I was needed at the liquor store. I felt bad that I couldn't keep working weekends for Dena, but in the end the liquor store job meant I had more money in my pocket to fulfill my binging habit ... and right now that trumped everything.

KEEPING BUSY

I will never forget the first time I met Warren. I was working an afternoon shift at the flower shop, and this nice looking man walked in. He was wearing a sharp-looking suit, and he really caught my eye. He was quite friendly while I took his information for a flower delivery. I assume he was getting flowers for his girlfriend. He told me that he knew Dena and asked me to say hello to her. The next day when I came to work, I asked Dena about him. She blushed a bit and said she just knew him from coming into the store. I figured he was probably ten years older than me. He came into the store a few more times after that, and he was always very chatty, almost a little flirty I thought. I wasn't used to that. I knew I wasn't overweight anymore, but to have a good-looking guy acknowledge me was flattering. I left it at that for two reasons: first he was in a relationship, and second he was much older than me. Oh right ... I had a boyfriend too! I wrote the encounters off just as an opportunity to see a "hot-looking" and stylish guy every once in a while.

September 1992 – Classes began at SIAST (Saskatchewan Institute of Applied Science and Technology; now called Saskatchewan Polytechnic) and we would soon begin our clinical experiences. That meant we would learn skills at school and then have an opportunity to practice them at various health care facilities in Regina. My first clinical assignment was at Wascana Rehabilitation Centre. We started at 6:00 a.m. with an instructor meeting who reviewed our patient load. This was it, I finally had a chance to put my skills to work. Bed baths were the majority of our tasks the first week. We also had to complete care plans for our patients. These plans were quite detailed and required a significant amount of preparation. I remember working on them for many hours, often into the early morning to complete them. I was finding the workload to be quite heavy but was managing. Once I got to work with my patients, it was easy for me. I loved meeting people and helping them in any way that I could. I was for sure a people person.

I also loved my job at the liquor store. I was proud to say that I worked there. Everyone on staff was very friendly. I was the youngest employee, but that didn't matter as I fit right in. I was never one to pick my friends by their age. If we got along, we got along. It was as simple as that. Because of my busy schedule at school and the liquor store, I was only able to work a few odd hours here and there at the flower shop. I tried to cover shifts for Dena whenever my schedule allowed, but eventually I had to resign from that job. Dave and I were still dating, but I didn't see as much of him either because of how busy I was between school and work.

And then there was my eating disorder. I can't forget about that. I continued to binge and purge, but the frequency had decreased because my life was so busy. That being said, the amount I would consume within a binge moment increased. I couldn't eat five chocolate bars during class or at the liquor store without anyone noticing. So when I did binge, I felt like I needed to make up for all the missed opportunities during the day. It was rational to me.

Even though my weight was still about the same, I began to fuss over the way clothes made me feel. I became more aware of the tightness of waistbands and the feel of clothes against my skin. As a result, I began using weigh scales more frequently. I knew if I had gained two pounds just by the way my work pants fit. I fluctuated between 115 and 122 pounds. My "bloated feeling" also depended on what time of the month it was … Period time was the worst. I felt like a fat pig, and I hated having to squeeze into my workpants. I only had two pair of workpants, both size six, but because they were different styles they fit a little differently. So I dressed accordingly. If I was having a "bloated day", my mood instantly spiraled downward. How I felt in my skin each morning would determine my mood for the day. In turn, I had a separate wardrobe for my "not-a-fat-pig" days. My mood was always better on those days.

I also seemed to be getting more colds. My immune system was not like it used to be. Granted, I was a smoker, but only a casual one at that time. I had not talked to my parents about my bulimia for quite some time. I don't think they really knew what to say about it … so they didn't say much.

Now that I had a little extra spending money, I could afford to buy more binge food. The cashier at the corner store made a comment that caught me off guard one day, "I don't know how you can eat all of these chocolate bars and stay so skinny." I didn't blame her one bit for saying that. The chocolate bars were three for ninety-nine cents, so I would often buy fifteen at once and then be at the corner store twenty-four hours later buying more. A concern crossed my mind. What if the cashier said something about my junk food purchases to my sister or dad? They often went to the same corner store to buy their cigarettes. The liquor store was in the same strip mall, so many of my co-workers also went to the corner store to buy snacks. I began to fret about my purchases. That created additional anxiety for me, but I was able to stay in check without medication despite my ever-changing moods. I was stronger than that. As long as I wasn't "found out" by anyone, things were still good.

I stepped up my creativity, in regards to hiding my eating disorder. There were so many recent changes in my life that my disorder had to adapt to the changes as well. Stopping the behavior was not an option. It never even crossed my mind to stop. I was fine with discovering a new way to adapt. "Hi, my name is Andrea, and I am a bulimic," could have easily been my motto. I didn't think I had a problem. Bulimia was just as normal and necessary to me as breathing.

A "normal" person eats when they are hungry. Your stomach may let you know this by "growling". For someone with an eating disorder it's different. If you are an *overeater*, you ignore the signals from your body that tell you that you have eaten enough. You eat whether you are hungry or not. You may love the taste of food, but sometimes that doesn't even matter. *Anorexics*, often get a "high" from the empty feeling in their stomachs. The restriction feels good. In the case of *bulimics*, at least for me, it was somewhat a combination of these other two eating disorders. I began the road to an eating disorder by restricting my intake. I "will-powered" myself to the extreme, much like an anorexic. Then, after not being able to handle the restriction anymore, I started binging just like an overeater. But here's the difference. When I got so emotionally overwhelmed with guilt after an eating binge, I needed to get rid of the food almost as quickly as it went down. Even though there are some differences, I learned that we all have these behaviors to fill some sort of emptiness in our souls. The only person who knows what is missing from their life is the person that is hurting. Hopefully, those that suffer from an eating disorder can find a way to manage that emptiness before serious or permanent harm is inflicted.

THE ESCALATION CONTINUES

My bubbly personality became my trademark. My boss at the liquor store told me that many customers had mentioned that I was the friendliest cashier they had ever met. I guess I don't know that for a fact, but I did get a few direct compliments from customers. My manager was also impressed with my customer service skills. I really enjoyed the job, it was fun and I got to meet many new people as it was very busy store.

My exams were in full swing at school and although I found my personal schedule hectic, I was doing well in school. I hoped all my hard work would pay off. Someday, I would be able to help people with their mental health issues. My parents were proud, especially since I almost failed out a year ago. I kept to my room when I was doing my schoolwork and ate while I studied. My parents were usually downstairs so I used the bathroom upstairs by my room. I began buying food from a few different stores to avoid the awkward questions. I also hit the fast food drive-thru restaurants. I would grab my food at the window and then pull over and eat in the parking lot. A regular order was usually a couple of burgers, onion rings and a large milkshake to wash everything down. After I was done, I would walk into the restaurant and purge in their washroom. This system worked well for me. I got my food, ate without someone else around me, and threw up in privacy. Sometimes, I had to lie to my boyfriend when he would ask where I was … I can't even recall what I told him. It was so "second nature" for me to fib to him. I think I even started to believe some of my own lies. As I think about those dark years, it doesn't even sound like me. But it was me. All of those life choices I made somehow brought me to where I am today. I have to keep reminding myself of that so I don't continue to beat myself up about my past.

Another Christmas came and went. Much like the year before, my holiday season binges were no longer a source of stress. They were just part of my daily routine. The winter semester at school was here again, and I was another year older. I was excited about my new clinical placement and I was proud of my academic progress. However, I seemed to be catching every flu bug that was going around. Something was definitely going on with my immune system. I was also aware that my teeth were beginning to feel and look different. When I went to the dentist, I always seemed to leave with another appointment card for further work. I was often nervous when I walked into the dentist office and usually pondered, "Maybe I should just tell them that I am bulimic? Although I probably don't have to say anything because they'll figure it out once they look at my teeth. The tips of my teeth are starting to thin, so I'm sure the dentist will suspect something. Okay, forget it. I won't say anything unless they bring it up. That will save me some embarrassment." I could deal with a few fillings. No big deal. To be honest, I don't even know if I cared about my teeth. Obviously I didn't because I kept throwing up. The dentist suggested that I get a mouth guard to wear at night. I knew that I grinded my teeth since

I was a kid, and several friends had mouth guards, so I figured this was an okay recommendation. The plan was to get a mouth guard fitted at my next appointment. Thank God I had dodged another medical bullet.

Mentally, my baseline behaviors continued to worsen. I was in my own world and assumed things were just fine. My mom checked in with me occasionally to see how I was doing. She didn't come out and ask me if I was bulimic. I can only imagine being in her shoes. I always said I was doing okay, and I would change the subject very quickly by telling her about school. Even though I was buying more of my own binge foods, I'm sure my parents still noticed the large amounts of groceries we were going through. I remember on one occasion, my dad got really mad. He got home from the store with something he bought just for him. I don't remember what item of food it was, but I do recall him getting it out of the grocery bag and waving it in front of me. "You better stay away from this because it's for me!" he said sharply. I got really defensive and we started arguing. That clarified things for me pretty quickly. There was no doubt that I wasn't fooling my parents anymore. I once again would have to find a way to revamp my system. Now I really had to make sure that I bought all the food that I binged. That way, even if my dad knew I was throwing up, he wouldn't be as mad because it was coming out of my pocketbook and not his. I really didn't want to resort to stealing from my mom's purse anymore. God knows I had already done enough of that when I was younger. "I'm sorry, Mom." I decided again that I would try to "be good" and not practice my eating disorder. That was becoming my norm, part of the cycle I was in, but my pattern changed a bit this time around. I began "being good" for five days and then I would "be bad" for the next five days. Whether good or bad, it was enough to get me through my winter semester of school. I knew that psychiatric nursing was my calling, so I was focused on completing that goal. It was one of the few roles in my life in which I was very comfortable. Caring for patients seemed much easier than caring for myself.

I was set to begin a six week practicum in the spring of 1993. My instructor placed me at a residential home for sex offenders under the age of fourteen. All the offenders were male and so were the workers. My first day there was a disaster. I felt so intimidated by these "boys". I was sure that I could win them over with my bubbly personality and my feminine charm. That didn't work. One boy cornered me in the house when no one was around. "I bet I could punch your damn head in right now." The fear that ran through me was almost paralyzing. "I bet you could," I responded. "And what would that prove? That you can beat up a girl half your size?" He didn't bother me again, except for some subtle flirtations toward me later on. That placement taught me many lessons. I said to my instructor half way through my practicum, "Why did you place me at such a challenging facility?" He responded, "Because I knew you needed to toughen up."

Physically speaking, my immunity continued to be challenged. At my worst, when I was purging twenty to thirty times a day, my ability to fight off ailments was depleted. When you add emotional stress to the equation, this habit was exhausting. I was experiencing a lot of heartburn and stomach aches. I often felt achy and flu-ish. My doctor wanted to check my esophagus after I told him about my "problem". Luckily it was fine. Of course, like before, I was mostly happy because that meant I could continue my addiction. I hadn't done any damage yet, so I may as well keep going was how I thought.

Since I hadn't been feeling well for a couple of weeks, I missed some school. I decided to tell my instructor about my bulimia. I was not prepared for what he told me. His response was for me to seriously think about dropping out of nursing in order to get better. I was instantly mad at him. "How dare he judge me just because I have an eating disorder," I thought. I told my parents what was going on, although I wasn't completely honest with them about how many times I was throwing up each day. I reassured them that I was well enough to continue my nursing course. I was determined to prove to everyone, that even though I had a "minor addiction", that I could still complete my nursing program. Having an addiction didn't mean that I was stupid. I guess that attitude saved me in one way because I completed my practicum. My instructor continued to check in to make sure I made up for my absenteeism. My marks were in the high-eighties after finals were complete. I was very proud of myself. I was going to do this!

August 1993 – I got a letter in the mail stating that I had been placed in Yorkton to begin my last year of school. I was scared. I had never been away from home for an extended period. I phoned some of my classmates to see where they were going. One of them was placed in Yorkton too. We decided to get an apartment together. The placement was for three and a half months starting after the Labour Day weekend. My boyfriend would probably miss me, but I was okay with that. I planned to continue working at the liquor store on weekends during the semester. Before the practicum began, a regular liquor store customer said to me, "Gee Andrea, you should try out for Miss Saskatchewan Roughrider this year. I think you would have a really good chance of winning." I didn't know what to say because I didn't think I was pretty enough for the competition. My first impression was that the title would be mostly based on looks and not personality or intelligence. However, after telling a few friends about the idea, they convinced me to get a sponsor and enter the contest. I had about six weeks until the competition weekend.

Classes began in Yorkton with my friend. We rented a cozy apartment close to the mall. We bought separate groceries and split the rest of the bills. I only binged and purged a few times a week because I was trying to "lose those extra few pounds" before the Miss Roughrider competition. My practicum was going well. I interned at an abilities center, which I enjoyed. I worked with wonderful individuals with various mental challenges. I remember being in the moment and genuinely caring for these people. My roommate wasn't aware that I was bulimic, and I wanted to keep it that way. It made things difficult at times. When she would go out, I knew I had a limited amount of time to have my small feast. The toilet was new so that reduced my stress.

The weekend arrived for the Saskatchewan Roughrider competition. I borrowed a dress from my sister. I had lost about ten pounds in six weeks for the event. There were about thirty other girls in the contest. They were all very pretty. We were all introduced at the luncheon. My parents attended with me. After the luncheon, each contestant was asked a question pertaining to football. I felt pretty good about my answers. The judges would announce the winner at the Labour Day game. All of us wore Roughrider sweatshirts and white sweats. We paraded onto the field at halftime. And the winner was ... not me. I don't even know why I shared this memory. It's not like it had a major impact on my life or anything, but I do know that I went right back to my old habits and gained the ten pounds back shortly afterwards. I guess maybe that's why I shared it.

My practicum was coming to an end, and Christmas was once again around the corner. My marks were in the nineties, and I really had a great educational experience at the Pine Unit in Yorkton. I was still going out with the same guy, but I could tell that the spark was fading. Dave was moving to Winnipeg in order to continue his schooling, and I can't really say that I was upset that we would be apart once again. We ended things shortly after he left for school. Over the years, we had some fun times and got fairly close with each other's families. I did care about him, but it was time to move on.

My last semester of nursing was finally here. I interned on the Acute Psychiatric Unit in Regina and also with Mental Health as a community mental health nurse. I also met a guy through some mutual friends. Vince and I became a couple shortly after. I was drawn by his looks and his easygoing nature. I didn't tell him too much about my eating habits right away as that would have definitely scared him off. I assumed not too many guys would want to know about an eating disorder this early in a relationship.

I had a successful final semester in school and had no doubt in my mind that I had chosen the right career path. I loved meeting people and was confident in my abilities. Helping people was what I wanted to do. Unfortunately, that still did not include me. I studied meticulously for my exams and did very well in all of them. The program had a final exam, and I also had to write a Provincial Registration Exam in order to receive my official nursing licence. I completed the program with a 92.4% average. I was proud of my accomplishment. Our nursing classmates voted me and another student as the graduation's master of ceremonies. We accepted the responsibility and were both honored to fulfill the role. I was excited about the ceremony because my family was coming, along with my new boyfriend. They were all very proud of me. My parents knew it had been a rough few years, but the rest of my family didn't know the severity of my eating disorder. Truthfully, the only one that really knew was me. I had completed my nursing course but had not yet overcome my eating disorder. That goal would turn out to be a lot harder to accomplish in the future than I could ever imagine.

Graduation night finally arrived, and I was both excited and nervous. All of the graduates were seated at the front of the hall. My friend and I rose to the podium to begin the ceremony. If I dare to say so, Bill and I did a pretty darn good job. We had so much fun up on stage and there was plenty of laughter. That made me happy. I was so caught up in the evening that I actually was able to remain in the moment. That was a big deal for me. Not being distracted by food and focusing on the task at hand without lies and deceit was a rarity. I received my diploma and once again it was an opportunity for a new beginning. Hopefully, this time without an eating disorder. I had a new boyfriend and a new career that awaited me. Who wouldn't be happy?

A FRESH START OR RUNNING
AWAY FROM MY PROBLEMS?

I always thought Monday mornings were special. That's the day that a person will start their new diet, stop smoking, start going to the gym, and whatever else that requires "self-discipline and willpower".

MONDAY'S

Today is Monday
The day I will stop
I've told myself
The weight will drop

I use my willpower
To gain some control
But then I'm tempted
By that oversized bowl

I try every Monday
But hope seems to fade
Just can't gain control
Is this how I'm made?

Defeated and scared
I go through my days
This has to be easier
There must be other ways

I struggle in my head
Every second of the day

Do I really want to stop?
Right now, I can't say

I accept the fact
I can't win this fight
There will be other Mondays
So for now, goodnight

I continued to work at the liquor store after graduation as there weren't many nursing opportunities in Regina. I got on the casual list at a long-term care facility, but that really wasn't an interest area of mine at the time. Socially, Vince and I were doing well. I tried explaining the problem I had with food to him, but I don't think he got it. In one way, I guess I could say that I had gained some control over my addiction. If a group of us was going out for a social evening, I would barely eat because I made the choice not to purge that evening. If anything, some friends may have thought I had some anorexic tendencies, but I wasn't real skinny, so that probably didn't make sense in their minds either.

Vince usually wanted to go to the bar with friends. I really didn't care to go mostly because I was insecure about our relationship in the bar scene due to my body image concerns. He was only my second boyfriend. Looking back, I guess I shouldn't have been so hard on myself. I was probably at my ideal weight and was fairly fit from attending aerobic classes, but I hated when my boyfriend would talk to other girls. And the more he drank, the friendlier he got with other girls. Sometimes he would go to the bar without me. I remember waiting by the phone for him to call me when he got home. I was a nervous wreck. I preferred when he would come over to my parents' to watch a movie or we would go to his parents' house and do the same. I got quite close with his parents. I felt like part of the family. Vince usually put himself first though. I now recognize that I didn't have enough self-worth to speak up and tell him that this seemed unfair. I was there when it was convenient for him. If his friends were busy on a Friday night he would call me and say, "I guess we can watch a movie tonight." I was maybe fourth on his list of friends to call, but when we were together, we did get along great. I just had to accept that I wasn't his first choice. He also went on two spring break trips with friends. Daytona Beach – tons of single women from all over the world. I wasn't stupid and I knew what spring break was all about. Did I care? Of course. Did I say anything? Of course not. God forbid that I would stand in the way of him having a good time or ask to tag along, or better yet, stand up for myself and have some self-dignity.

I was with Vince for about two years when my friend, Leanne, asked me if I wanted to go on a hot holiday to Florida. She worked for an airline and her sister also lived in Florida, so it would be fairly inexpensive. What a great opportunity. I built up my courage and asked my boyfriend for "permission". He had just gotten back from a boys' holiday so he didn't really care if I went. It was not like he was controlling, actually maybe even the opposite. Maybe he just didn't realize what he had with me, basically a girlfriend that let him do whatever he wanted whenever he wanted. Leanne booked our holiday; I couldn't believe we were going. I would miss my boyfriend, but I was definitely due for a girls' trip.

Leanne and I arrived in Orlando, and her sister picked us up from the airport. We got to her place on the beach, and the weather was gorgeous. The next morning we laid on the sand and soaked up the sun. Later, Leanne's sister wanted to drive to Fort Lauderdale to get some work done on her car. Even though the two of us just wanted to relax and tan we agreed to go along with her. We were driving along the coast for about twenty minutes when Leanne's sister decided to make a pit stop at a beach bar. She wanted to see if a guy she used to like was still bartending there. We went in, and there were just a few people inside. The guy she hoped to see wasn't there. As we were glancing around, we noticed two guys playing billiards. They were both very good looking and, of course, I was completely embarrassed by the way

I looked. I had showered before we left, but I had no makeup on and my hair was completely flat. My cheeks were sunburned, and I was wearing a tacky outfit that I had bought in Hawaii years ago. It was full of pineapples and grapes. Who wears stuff like that? I guess I did. Besides, I had no idea we would be running into "hot" looking guys at a beach bar anytime soon. The two guys soon noticed us sitting at the bar and asked us if we wanted to play pool with them. We decided why not and that we would go to Fort Lauderdale tomorrow instead. I quickly put some lipstick on, so that at least I wouldn't feel like a complete loser. The one guy was Italian and was very cute and funny. I thought for sure he would be interested in Leanne because she was also Italian and a bombshell. Ironically enough, he seemed to sway toward me and my fancy fruit-colored outfit from the eighties. What could he possibly see in me? Leanne had beautiful long hair and a body to kill. Anyway, we enjoyed our game of pool, and we talked and laughed. I think it was around 6:00 p.m. when they asked us if we wanted to meet them at a nightclub that evening. We enthusiastically accepted the invitation and drove home to change. I don't know what I was thinking. I had a boyfriend. Well, what harm could come from one night of partying with a couple of guys? As if Vince hadn't partied with other girls over the years.

We met them at the bar a few hours later. I had curled my hair, applied makeup, and put on a cute skirt and top. Tommy, the Italian, complimented me on my transformation. His friend, Trent, definitely took a liking to Leanne as well. We ordered some drinks and had a few dances. It was all very innocent, at least until a certain song came on. I will never forget that dance. Talk about seductive. Our bodies ended up getting closer and closer as the song went on. I remember thinking how this wasn't right for me to be feeling this way, but Tommy was so good at what he did (seducing)! Next thing I knew our lips met on the dance floor. Needless to say, we spent our entire week with Tommy and Trent.

I talked to my boyfriend a few times while in Florida. I told him we were having a great time, but I obviously left out the fact that I met Tommy. I felt guilty, but I was so hypnotized by the idea of Tommy liking me that I didn't want the week to end. I couldn't believe how quick our trip seemed to fly by. On our last night, Tommy offered to drive us to the airport the next day. I couldn't believe how sad I was to be leaving. I would never see this gorgeous guy who swept me off my feet again. I cried the whole way to the airport. Why was I feeling this way? I loved my boyfriend, or at least I thought I did. This was probably just a short fling that I would now have to keep secret. I figured I would eventually forget about this week with Tommy after I got back home. I had his number, and he said I could call him if I wanted. He respected the fact that I had a boyfriend and a whole different life back in Regina.

Our flight arrived about three hours late. My mom and dad were at the airport along with Vince. I gave him a big hug and kiss. He told me I looked amazing with my suntan. He drove me home in my car, which he had been driving while I was away. He offered to pick me up in the morning and take me to work. That was kind of out of character for him. As I fell asleep that night though, all I could think about was Tommy. Vince picked me up in the morning and took me to work. "I'll pick you up at lunch and we can go over to my place," he said. He was acting really strange. It was like he actually missed me. Maybe he realized what it feels like when your partner goes on a trip without you. We got to his place on my lunch break, and he was super-affectionate and even made me lunch. He took me back to work and then drove me home after I was done work as well.

A few days went by and Leanne called me. She had talked to Trent and he had a message for me. Tommy wanted me to call him. I debated if I should call or not. My boyfriend was treating me wonderfully these last few days. He even cancelled some plans with the guys to be with me. After thinking about it for a bit, I picked up my phone and found myself dialing Tommy's number. As soon as I heard his voice, it took me back to Florida. He told me that he missed me. I told him that I was thinking of him as well. We phoned each other almost every night after that.

I guess I haven't mentioned where I was at with my bulimia during this time. When we were in Florida I didn't binge or purge once. I was able to control the urge. As soon as I got back home I went right back to my old ways. I did tell Tommy that I was dealing with some personal issues, but that's all I said. One evening after Vince left my house, Tommy and I were chatting. He told me that he knew some people that worked at a mental health facility near him in Florida. He told me that they would like to interview me. I think my heart almost stopped. What was I going to do? I had my boyfriend, job, and family in Regina. Could I actually pack up and move away to live with a guy that I actually didn't really know that well? The idea was so out there, but I was intrigued by the thought. What would my parents say? What about my boyfriend? Like I said, Vince was acting like a different guy lately. He knew we had met some guys in Florida and partied together, but as if he hadn't done the same on his spring break trips.

I told Tommy that I needed some time to think about his offer. The thought of working in Florida seemed way too much like living in a fairy tale. I tried to stay focused in the moment, but found it hard not to stress about my dilemma. Tommy called a few days later to see what I had decided. I knew there was a bunch of paperwork that needed to be done in order to get a job in the United States. For now, I thought, I could tell Customs that I was vacationing and not mention anything about a job interview. Another major issue was that the State of Florida required out-of-state nurses to write a lengthy qualification exam that only Registered Nurses were eligible to write. The State of Florida did not acknowledge Registered Psychiatric Nurses as part of their health system. Despite all these hurdles, I was blinded by excitement.

The next thing I knew, I was booked on a flight to Florida and was leaving in one week. Tommy even wired me the money for the flight. Vince was shocked when I told him that I had an interview in Florida.

He couldn't believe it and said, "So, like what the hell will happen to us? You must have something going on with that Tommy guy. Why else would you want to go?" I lied through my teeth. I told him that Leanne's sister had set up the interview, and I would be staying with her. The next few days, Vince kept his distance, and I continued to chat with Tommy every night. The plan was to stay in Florida for only three days as I had to get back for work. When I arrived, Tommy was at the airport to greet me. All of the feelings rushed back. The next day, I met with the director of the mental health facility. He agreed that I was qualified for a job there and said they would hire me if I could get a working visa. I figured that was a minor technicality.

Tommy and I went out dancing later that evening. Boy was this "the life." I could live in a beautiful place, get a part-time job, and live with Tommy. I would stop my bulimic habits and get healthy again. A new place, a new identity, a fresh start. I landed back at Regina airport and just my mom was there to greet me. I called Vince the next day, which was difficult. I told him that I was going to take the job in Florida. He pretty much hung up on me. My parents were concerned too. "Ange, have you actually thought this through?" my mom asked. My dad definitely figured I was being way too spontaneous. I lied and told them I would be living with Leanne's sister. I did tell my mom about Tommy. I think she knew what was going on; Mom's aren't stupid. I put in my resignation at the liquor store. Wow … I really would be moving to Florida in three weeks! Vince was all over the map with his reaction. Rightfully so, I guess. I told him that I didn't want to break up with him and this was just something I needed to do for myself. Honestly, what was I thinking? I wanted to have "my cake and eat it too". My friends at work planned a going away party for me. Vince didn't come.

One night about three days before I was leaving, I ran into Vince at a pool hall. He approached me and asked if he could drive me home. I was pretty shocked considering he hadn't talked to me for days. On the way home, he told me that we should consider getting engaged! Vince was the furthest thing from a 'settle down' type of guy. So basically, he didn't want me to go to Florida and would marry me if I stayed? I told him that I knew he was just saying that to keep me in Regina. Nothing else was mentioned after that. The next day I went to his place to say goodbye to his parents. This was difficult as I had grown close to his parents over the past couple years. His dad, Melvin, didn't want me to go. I found out later that Melvin told a friend that he thought of me as a daughter. Vince took me home, and we had a pretty intense goodbye moment. I started to cry, wondering if I had made the right choice. It was too late now. All of the arrangements were made. Well not really, but that's what I told everyone. I cried all night wondering about several things. Did Vince really want to marry me? Was Tommy really as great as he seemed? I guess I would find out.

My mom and dad took me to the airport early in the morning. My best friend Wendy showed up too. I hugged Wendy and my parents. There were more tears. It was very hard to say goodbye. I landed in Florida, and there was Tommy. I ran to him and figured everything would be okay now. We got to his place, and I got settled in. I called my mom and dad. They didn't have caller identification on their phone, which saved some explaining. "The weather is beautiful here," I shared. This was going to be awesome. Tommy, his roommate Eric, and I had a few drinks to celebrate my arrival. Tommy and I talked about our future together. He reassured me that if I ever needed to fly home for something important that he would take care of things. How could I ask for a better guy?

The next day Tommy went to work, and I decided to go out and buy some groceries. Just like that my cravings crept up on me again. I went straight from the grocery store to a fast food joint. I ordered enough burgers for a whole family and wolfed them down in my vehicle. I then walked in and headed straight for the bathroom. I did it all so robotically, like it was exactly what I was supposed to do. This continued on for days. All of my problems had followed me to Florida. I hadn't even been to the immigration office in Orlando yet, and I had already been there for about a week. I decided I'd better go the next day. When I got to the office, I was surprised to see an extremely long lineup of people. What had I gotten myself into? I can honestly say now that I probably had no intention of working in Florida because I knew it would be near impossible to secure all the legal paperwork. Eight hours later, I was given a handful of phone numbers related to transferring my nursing marks. I left quite discouraged by the red tape that stood in my way.

I got back to Tommy's and thought I'd better check in with my parents. I told them I was getting things in order, but it would take a while. "I thought you had all that stuff figured out before you left?" my dad questioned. More dishonesty followed on my part. I also told them that I had to stay at Tommy's for a bit because my friend was having financial problems. I'm not sure how that went over, but really what could they do about it from Regina. There was some good news though, my sister Kim and my best friend Wendy had decided to come visit me. When they arrived we spent time tanning at the pool and went out dancing. I still hadn't given much effort to acquiring a working visa, but I did get my marks transferred. It wasn't long before I was running out of money. I had been there three weeks and my funds were dwindling away. I continued to secretly buy food to binge and purge, which didn't help matters. Tommy had no idea.

I don't know exactly when I started noticing another side to Tommy, but I did. On one occasion, he phoned from work and said he would appreciate lemon pepper chicken for supper. While I was cooking, I noticed that he didn't have all the ingredients in the kitchen, so I made him honey garlic chicken instead not thinking it was a big deal. I was wrong, he made it into a very big deal, "I told you I wanted lemon pepper and that's what you should have made me." I was shocked at how upset he got over something fairly trivial. It was the first time he had raised his voice at me, and I guess it caught me off guard. His roommate heard and told me later in private not to worry about it. Tommy also didn't want to go out very much. I guess that was understandable as he was working every day, while I thought I was on an extended holiday. My problems definitely didn't go away in Florida like I thought they would. I felt very defeated once again.

I phoned Vince a couple of times to see how he was doing. He still thought I was staying with my girlfriend. We talked civilly to each other, but it was usually brief. On Friday, September 13, a friend from Regina called to let me know that Vince's dad had passed away suddenly. My heart sank, and I instantly wanted to go home. I called my parents and told them what happened in between my sobs. I called the airline to see if I could use my open ticket. It was exactly one month since I had arrived, so I was able to make the switch for fifty dollars because it was for a funeral. I then phoned Vince and offered my condolences. I told him I was coming home in a couple days. I then told Tommy what had happened. He wasn't too happy that I had already booked my flight. Wendy wasn't leaving for another week, but she insisted that I go to Regina, and she would spend some time in Orlando. Tommy gave me the silent treatment for the next day and a half. The only thing that he said was that I just can't run home every time someone dies. I guess he had forgotten his promise to fly me home whenever I needed. He drove us to Orlando, dropping Wendy off at her hotel and me at the airport. I gave him a hug before I boarded the plane and told him that I would call. At the time, I had all intentions of coming back to Florida as I only brought a few of my clothes with me, but things changed.

BACK TO REALITY AND MORE TURMOIL

I was so happy to see my parents at the Regina airport four hours later. I cried when I saw them. We got to their house, and I freshened up. I remember my heart pounding on the drive over to Vince's house with my parents. All I could hear in my head were those words Melvin said to me, "I don't want you to go, Andrea. I wish you would stay." We knocked on the door and Vince's brother-in-law answered. We exchanged hugs and made our way downstairs. Vince was standing there, and I just held him and cried. I was so sorry for his loss and everything I had done that he didn't know about. I hadn't seen his mom yet, so I went upstairs. When she saw me she just started bawling, and I comforted her with a hug. My mom and dad stayed for a bit, but I told them that I would come home later. Vince and I sat on the couch beside each other and recalled memories of his dad. No questions were asked about Florida, and I didn't offer any details. I held him and stroked his hair. I was so overwhelmed with guilt and shame, I just kept crying. I thought maybe this was Mel's way of telling me I had made a mistake. The funeral was the next day, and Vince's mom wanted me to sit with the family. Vince said that was okay.

The funeral was kind of a blur to me. Until then, I don't think I had ever cried so much in my life. I think our friends were shocked to see me there. Melvin was going to be buried in his hometown about two hours away on the following day. I was asked to come along and spend the night at Vince's grandma's house. Of course I went. We stood around the gravesite after the burial and toasted a shot of vodka to Mel. I was glad to be there for such an intimate celebration of his life. That night, Vince and I spent time reconnecting. I knew he was very vulnerable, but that didn't matter. I just kept telling myself that I had screwed up. When I got to my parents' the next day, I asked Mom if I could "come home". I knew I had made a terrible mistake, and I hoped it wasn't too late to fix things. I can hear my mom as if it were yesterday, "You didn't make a mistake; you made a choice. We all need to make choices in life because they give us direction. There may be consequences to deal with because of the choices made, but that is all part of life … and, of course you can come home dear."

Soon after I had to deal with my "new life" back in Florida. I called Tommy and told him I thought it would be best if I stayed in Regina. I tried to explain to him why. "Remember that problem that I told you I had, well I am not doing so good. I really think I need to go to the doctor. I am so sorry, and I will really miss you." The receiver was silent. I suppose my decision came as a shock to him. I'm not sure if I really understood what was going on myself. Actually, that's probably not quite right, it was probably more like denial. I think I knew deep down exactly what was going on, and it had nothing to do with my eating disorder. I was overwhelmed with guilt and decided that I wanted Vince back. We had gotten closer than ever before over the last few days, and I figured that if I just moved back our relationship would blossom. I asked my friend to send my belongings back to Regina from Florida. I didn't know what else to say to Tommy. He was probably wondering what the hell just happened. Later, I called the manager of the liquor store and begged for my job back. Luckily, he said yes. Things would be okay, or so I thought.

The next day I saw Vince. I told him that I had made a big mistake by leaving for Florida, and that I was staying home. "I hope you're not staying because of me," was his response. I said that things hadn't worked out job-wise, and it would be too difficult to get a Florida nursing licence. That wasn't a complete lie, but more importantly, I wanted us to be together. As I am writing this story today, I am puzzled by the fact that so far it seems like all my focus has been on everyone else but myself. I had this serious, secretive eating disorder issue, and yet I didn't think it was that big of a problem (denial is the first stage they say).

The next few months were absolutely horrible. I was phoning Vince nonstop. I actually came straight out and told him that I wanted him back. "You broke my heart," was all he said. I could not accept it, or picture my life without him. I soon started back at work as I had a nine hundred dollar phone bill to pay off. Thank God, I had my parents to live with. Of course, during this whole time, I was spending loads of money on my food addiction. I was also going out on the weekends with my friends, many of which were Vince's friends too. I was still trying desperately to get him back and was overcome with guilt because of all the lies that I had told him. His cold shoulder made me want him more than ever. One night, we all met at a friend's house before heading to the bar. I wore a revealing top hoping that Vince would notice. The other guys made a complimentary comment and Vince agreed. I thought this was wonderful. I figured we would get to the bar, dance a bit, we would make up, and I would go home with him. This didn't happen.

Unfortunately, this night would turn out to be a disaster. The bar was packed, but I saw a few friends so I went and hung out with them while trying to keep track of Vince's whereabouts. All of a sudden, my eyes found him, talking face to face with a tall blonde. He had his arm around her in an intimate manner. His friends were with me, and they all watched too. They told me just to forget about him. I couldn't do that. I immediately started crying and ran out of the bar. I sat down on the floor in the lobby. I had my house keys in my hand. The next thing I knew, I was scratching up my leg with the keys. My friend Leanne found me. She got me up and offered to take me home. Vince showed up as we were leaving. Leanne started yelling at him and told him to just leave me alone from now on. We left.

When I got home, I was a mess. Everything seemed foggy. Like I was having a bad dream, and I just needed to wake up for everything to be okay. My sister Kim was home. I told her what happened, or at least tried to, while freaking out. She noticed my leg. I told her what I did. I don't know how I got to sleep that night, but when I woke up the next morning, I felt even worse. I was having trouble accepting the consequences of my choices. Kim was very worried about me. She phoned the psychiatrist on call at the hospital and about two hours later I was packing my suitcase to be admitted to the psychiatric unit on which I worked occasionally. Kim told my mom and dad that it was for the best, and they drove me there.

I arrived onto the unit and thought, "What the hell am I doing? I am probably going to know half of the staff." Oh well. I knew I needed some help. Unfortunately, I hadn't realized yet that the main cause for my turmoil wasn't the fact that I was no longer with Vince, but instead that I had a much deeper and more serious mental health issue. I wasn't ready to own up to that yet. I hardly shared anything about my eating disorder with the medical staff. When I did, I minimized the problem. So, I was put on some antidepressants to deal with my depression-like symptoms.

A few friends came by to visit the next morning. Just after lunch, the nurse told me I had another visitor. It was Vince. I don't know if I wanted to hug him or kick him. I asked him why he came. "I still care about you," he said. Then I got mad. How could he say that after what he did? Then I thought to myself, what if he knew what I had done? That made me feel guilty. He said goodbye and told me to phone him when I got out of the hospital. I think I was home about two days later.

I was encouraged by my doctor to see a counsellor about my bulimia, so I took his advice. I was given the number of a doctor in Saskatoon who treated patients with eating disorders. I was scheduled for treatment in one week. I told Vince that I was going, and I told my boss that I would need a little time off work. Before I knew it, I was checking into yet another psychiatric unit.

The doctor introduced himself. Right off the get-go, I didn't care for him. He was the type who didn't fall for crying and the "poor me" thing. I was given daily menu choices along with the doctor's recommendation to throw up at least one of those meals. What kind of therapy was this? How was I supposed to stop purging if they are telling me to vomit after eating my meal? Despite my doubts, I tried following the program laid out for me.

We had nightly group sessions where everyone got a chance to share their story. One girl had been through the treatment program five times already. She was hospitalized several times because of her anorexic body weight. Another girl was an overeater. Besides the three of us, the rest of the group had some other type of mental illness. I ate my two meals a day and then ate my one planned "binge-purge meal." It seemed weird, but that's what I did. Halfway through week two, I convinced the doctor that I was better. I'm pretty sure he knew I was trying to con him, but he knew that there was no point keeping me there if I wasn't ready to change my thinking and self-harming behaviours. I had lost about ten pounds while I was there ... surprise, surprise.

I took the bus back to Regina. My parents were both at work when I got to the bus depot. I called Vince, and he came and picked me up. He asked how I was doing, and I said fine. That was it. I was sure that he was dating the tall blonde, but he just didn't want to admit it. I started back to work and back to my purging ways just as quickly. All that treatment was down the drain, or should I say toilet?

I remained single for a while and slowly started getting over Vince. My friends were a big help in that process. I had only worked a few nursing shifts since I had graduated. Like I said, there weren't any permanent positions open and quite frankly, I don't know if I was ready for that type of responsibility at this point in my life. Instead, my friends and I partied the summer away. I either ate a lot in private or barely ate when I was in the public eye. I still had my most severe binges at home when nobody was around. For example, I would eat two birthday cakes, a two-litre of ice cream, a couple bags of cookies, and around ten chocolate bars in about two hours; obviously, not all at once, but in successive binging and purging sessions. I often had to take a break before throwing up because I occasionally ate so much that my stomach hurt. It hurt so much from being so full that I could barely walk. But boy, did I feel better after I got rid of it all. I would eat absolutely anything; it didn't matter. I bought my own food because I had wasted so much of my parents' food in the past. I knew that wasn't fair to them. Also, it helped keep my dad off my back and from them figuring out how much I was eating. My parents did ask me from time to time how I was doing. I always told them fine. I'm sure they knew that I was lying, but what could they do ... I was supposedly a mature adult now who could make her own decisions of what was best.

TIME TO MOVE ON

The summer was coming to an end, and my girlfriends and I had so much fun. I was running to the corner store early one morning for some snacks, literally just after getting out of bed, and I heard a voice say, "Hi." I turned around and saw a tall, muscular, good-looking guy. It was Warren, the same "older" guy that I had met a few years ago at the flower shop. By the time we finished chatting, he asked me if he could give me a call sometime. I said, "Sure." I was a bit dumbfounded, as I looked like crap, no makeup, and he wanted to go out on a date. I gave him my number and he said that he would call me in a couple weeks after he got back from a business trip. I told my friend and she was so excited for me. I had my doubts, "He's probably not even going to remember to call, and why would he want to go out with me?" I told myself not to get my hopes up.

About two weeks later, the phone rang, and it was Warren. I couldn't believe he actually called. We made plans for the following night as I had a staff gathering. I figured he was about ten years older than me, and I was right. I was twenty-five and he was thirty-five. He had that salt and pepper hair, which I found very attractive. He dressed sharply, and everything was brand name. Warren was a pharmaceutical rep, which meant he was smart and charismatic too. We hit it off right away. My co-worker girlfriends thought he was totally hot. We left the party, and he invited me over to his place. His house was a beautiful character home. He kept it very clean and neatly decorated. I ended up spending the night. What was I thinking? I wasn't that type of girl (or was I?). Oh well, it happened. He promised to call me in a few days. I called my friend, and she wanted to know every detail. Maybe this was the start of something new and fabulous (again) … I hoped anyway.

Warren and I got together a few more times before he called me one morning and suggested that we go for coffee. Our relationship wasn't real serious at this point as it had only been a couple of weeks since we began dating. I was just thrilled that a guy like him would want to be with me. Seriously, I was still driving my dad's old van. I was a psychiatric nurse, but worked at the liquor store more than I did at the hospital. I had a few new outfits in my wardrobe, but I always bought them on sale. Warren on the other hand ... well, I think his skincare products cost more than all my clothes put together. He spent his days meeting with doctors and went to symphonies in the evening with clients, yet somehow he was interested in me. I was very flattered. This all went through my head on the way to the coffee shop. When I arrived he had already gotten us a table, and he looked great. We started with small talk and then the conversation moved in a more serious direction. He started out by saying that his job was very demanding and that he was always on the road. In a roundabout way he told me that he couldn't give me a serious commitment. I remember getting up from the table and saying, "Okay then. No problem, give me a call sometime if you want."

I didn't hear from Warren for a couple of days. I had just finished a dayshift at the liquor store and walked to my vehicle. There was a note on the windshield that read: *Would you like to come to my place for supper tonight? Call me when you get home, Warren.*

"All right ... why not?" I thought. I went over, and we enjoyed each other's company, but I left it up to him to call me after that date. He seemed more committed to having a relationship, so we had some good times together. He introduced me to sushi, the symphony, and he had some nice friends. I always felt though, that I had to be "the girlfriend that he wanted me to be", and that I couldn't be myself. Perhaps it was the ten year age difference? Warren also said that he did not want to have kids. I almost had myself convinced that I didn't want kids either. That was weird, because as I look back now, I know I had always wanted kids someday. Once again, I had fallen into a pattern of putting someone else's needs before mine.

I told Warren about my eating disorder once our relationship became a bit more serious. He wasn't shocked. He said his ex-girlfriend had the same problem and that was pretty much the end of the conversation. So, I continued eating and throwing up knowing full well that my boyfriend was aware. Sometimes I even purged at his place, but I still made sure it wasn't obvious. At home, things were status quo. I loaded up with food and went up to my room to chow down. It had become so natural for me that I didn't realize I had a problem. I didn't have a lot of money, so occasionally I continued to steal money from my mom's purse. That was hard for me to write. I'm going to take a break now.

A COSTLY ADDICTION IN MORE WAYS THAN ONE

I guess while I'm being completely honest, I should share something else. For me, food was a drug, and I looked very forward to my binges. That's often all I thought about. Did I have enough money to buy binge food? When can I find some time to be alone so no one will interrupt me? These thoughts constantly raced through my head. Again, it was often very hard to be in the moment. As I think of that time now, I am ashamed of how I took advantage of my family, and how I stole from my mom. As tears roll down my cheeks, I ask for your forgiveness Mother. I also continue to try and forgive myself for this dishonesty. I love you, Mom.

Okay, a few deep breaths, and I will continue. Back to my relationship with Warren. Like I mentioned, I wasn't always myself around him. I guess I never really was with any of my boyfriends. I based my feelings on how they felt. If my boyfriend was in a good mood, then so was I. Sadly, if he was in a bad mood then my day was ruined too. I never allowed myself to really feel my own feelings, especially when I was with a boyfriend. For the most part, I was numb to my own emotions.

Warren and I had been dating for almost two years. There was a connection between us, but it definitely wasn't love. He had no idea who I really was or what my intimate thoughts were, and I'm sure he didn't care to find out. Truthfully, I probably didn't care either. I remember thinking to myself, "Why am I still dating this guy? I can't have a future with someone that doesn't know the real me. And I think I do want to have kids someday." The next weekend we went out of town for one of Warren's pharmaceutical conventions. I decided that I would just try to be myself on the trip, whether he liked it or not. I enjoyed meeting some really nice people, but otherwise the weekend was a disaster. The car ride home was very quiet. Warren dropped me off at my parents' house, and I barely said goodbye.

When we talked later, I told him that I didn't think things would work out for us. I would never be the person that he was looking for. He wanted to keep trying, so I agreed to see how things go. This was a big deal in my life. I had actually acknowledged the fact that I was pretending. It may not sound like much, but it was for me. Our relationship lasted for about another two months. I couldn't do it anymore. I also told him that I wanted to have kids someday too. That was enough to end our relationship. I told Warren that I was tired of trying to be the person he wanted me to be. I said, "Why don't you go on the Internet and type in the kind of woman you are looking for … You might get what you want, she'll be well-educated, intelligent, independent, and a great golfer, but will you love each other? Hell, she may even worship the ground you walk on … but sorry that's not me." Warren called me a few times after that, but as far as I was concerned, our relationship was dead.

My mother, once again, was there for me. Mom said she knew Warren wasn't the guy for me soon after we started dating, but she also knew that I had to figure that out on my own. I told my mom that the next guy I dated was going to love to dance and make me laugh. Or at least, that's what I was hoping to find in a partner.

WAS THIS FINALLY MR. RIGHT?

A few months went by and life carried on. Go to work, have some good laughs, come home, eat a bunch of food, throw up just as much, get dressed, and go out with some friends. That's what I did. One particular night my friend Wendy and I went to the bar and ran into an old friend. Angela and I chatted for a bit and then she pointed out her husband to me from across the bar. He was with a few other guys, but one of them caught my eye. The night was so much fun, with the girls just dancing up a storm! I truly loved dancing. It made me feel so alive; I could just be myself. I wasn't trying to impress anyone, I just danced to the beat and had a great time. After an hour or so, as Wendy and I were getting ready to leave, my friend Angela approached me. She told me that her husband's friend had been asking about me. That was cool because I was curious about him too. She introduced us, and we briefly chatted. I remember his smile and his sense of humor. However, it was closing time so Wendy and I left. I told my mom the next day that I ran into Angela and that she had introduced me to this guy. I recall telling Mom, "I don't even remember his name, but there was something about him. And he was funny too, but he doesn't live in Regina so I doubt that I will run into him again."

A couple of weeks went by, and I sort of forgot about that boy I had met. Actually, I guess I didn't really forget, but I figured we wouldn't meet again. That weekend, I planned to attend a "stagette" for my friend Tanya. The girls all met at a restaurant for a few drinks. While we were there, I ran into Angela again as she was a mutual friend of the bride-to-be as well. "Hey, Andrea," she said to me, "Remember my hubby's friend I introduced you to? Well, guess what, he's in town again, and the guys are probably going to meet up with us at the bar tonight." That caught my attention. I didn't want to get too excited as maybe he wouldn't even remember me. After nine years of dating and a few relationship disasters, I had grown pretty cautious of throwing my heart out there in any vulnerable manner. Maybe my "Mr. Right" just didn't exist.

We got to the dance club a few hours later and sure enough "the boy" and the other guys were there. Angela reintroduced us. His name was Mick. After chatting for a while he asked me to dance. We were having fun on the dance floor when he asked me if I wanted a drink. I said sure. Mick spun around and grabbed a couple full beers that the waitress had just put on the ledge for someone else. He handed one to me and said, "Cheers!" I burst out laughing as I couldn't believe he had the nerve to do something so impulsive. A couple minutes later a girl came looking for the beers. Mick went over to her and said something, she laughed. He handed her ten bucks and she was a good sport about it. I thanked him for the dance, and we both went back to hang out with our separate group of friends. Wendy and I had to leave earlier than the other girls, so once again I left feeling a little curious about this new boy named Mick.

The next morning I told my mom that I ran into "that guy" again and that we had so much fun dancing. She was happy to see that I was considering the dating scene again. I wondered if I would ever see Mick again, let alone date him. That evening I came out of the shower and my dad had a message for me, "Some Nick or Mick guy called and left a number for you to call him back." Wow, that was exciting news. Mick answered when I called. He was staying at a friend's house in Regina for a few days and was wondering if I wanted to go out for a drink or movie. I hadn't been to a movie for a while, so we decided to do both.

I remember counting the minutes before he picked me up. I was nervous and excited. The doorbell rang. I opened the door and introduced him to my mom because she of course was right beside me to check Mick out. My dad followed close behind. After some quick introductions we were off on our first date. We chatted on the way, mostly about how much fun we had the other night at the dance club. Mick said that he asked my friend Angela for my number after I did my "Cinderella disappearing act" from the bar. I was glad she gave it to him. We got to the theatre and tried to decide on a movie. He, like most guys, wanted to see an action show and I wanted to see *Notting Hill*, a comedy/romance "chick flick". When we got to the front of the line, the cashier asked what movie we were going to and Mick said, "Hi ... well, I want to see the James Bond movie, but she wants a chick flick, so we'll have two tickets to *Notting Hill* please." I remember thinking how sweet that was. I didn't want to get my hopes up, but I really thought this guy was different than all my ex-boyfriends. Who knows? Maybe this was finally Mr. Right? As I write this, I am struck by how most of my energy seemed to center around finding Mr. Right. That basically tells me just how sick I was. The most important thing should have been my health and self-worth, but I still wasn't at that point in my life quite yet.

Back to our date. The movie was romantically funny, and we had a few good laughs. We left the theater and went to a lounge for a drink. For the most part, our conversation was pretty superficial since we were just getting to know each other. I found out exactly where he lived, a few things about his family, and that he was a teacher in Langenburg. I shared my background, basically that I was a nurse, working casually, and that I worked at the liquor store too. We had a few more laughs, but before we knew it was after midnight. It then struck me that he still had a two and a half hour drive to get home and then had to work in the morning. He drove me home and walked me up to the front door. He said something about "talking soon", but I was a bit distracted with wondering if he was going to kiss me or not. He said goodnight and walked back to his car. I really would have enjoyed a kiss, but that was okay. It was still a fun evening. Maybe he was just trying to be a gentleman, so I hoped he would call soon.

Two days later, and I hadn't heard from Mick yet. I called Angela for some advice. She figured I should just call him and invite him to Tanya's wedding. I built up my courage and dialed his number. A voice answered that didn't sound like his. "Just a minute, I'll get him," said the voice. Mick came on and my heart started pounding. I said hello and told him who it was. I was relieved that it seemed like he was glad I called. After about ten minutes of chatting, I threw the question out there, "So, I was wondering if you would like to go to Tanya's wedding with me?" To my delight, he said yes. The wedding was in two weeks. Then to my surprise, he returned the invite and asked me to join him at his best friend's wedding in Langenburg. The Langenburg wedding wasn't for another six weeks. To me that was a good sign that we had a date that far in advance. We chatted a little bit longer, and I found out he had two roommates. We laughed some more, then said goodbye after promising to talk again soon.

Workwise, I started getting more shifts on the acute psychiatric unit in Regina. Yes, the same place I had briefly been a patient at a few years earlier. I had gotten some casual work at a nursing home too, which I enjoyed. I soon found my nursing skills, which I hadn't used for quite some time, coming back to me. I felt my confidence growing. The psychiatric unit was very emotionally draining, but I really enjoyed it. I was on the casual list for work, so the phone rang at all hours of the night, but I usually went in. I had some friends on staff, and we would go down to the cafeteria at lunch. I would always get the salad bar. I thought it would look like I'm eating healthy. I considered the salad bar "safe" foods even though most of it was loaded with ranch dressing, and I usually had plenty of potato salad. I always skipped the deep fried food just to avoid any suspicions. However, I still waited to see which washroom everyone was using after lunch and then picked a different one. I can't believe I never fainted at work due to low blood-sugar levels. Minutes later, I was in a patient's room counselling them. It all just seemed normal to me. Not too many people outside of my family really knew I had this secret. Actually, it was more than a secret. I was living a life completely full of lies. I don't think I really knew how I felt at times, because I was often mentally numb from binging and purging.

Mick and I chatted several times after I invited him to the wedding. Actually there were two weddings on that weekend. The first wedding was at 1:00 p.m. with a small reception afterwards and then the second wedding was at 3:30 p.m. with a full supper and dance to follow. Mick was coming into Regina on Friday and he asked me to go out for supper that evening. I couldn't wait to see him again. He picked me up and met my parents again. We had an enjoyable night that was filled with interesting conversation. We were really getting to know each other. I loved his sense of humor, and I think he even thought I was funny. He drove me home and this goodbye was definitely better than the first one. We shared a kiss; it felt so right. We thanked each other for the fun evening and were excited about tomorrow's weddings. I was so happy that night that I can't even remember if I kept that meal down; maybe, but I have my doubts.

The next morning I got my hair done for the day and loved it. I had a beautiful black velvet dress on and couldn't wait for Mick to arrive. When he did, I'm pretty sure his eyes popped out of his head. "You look great!" he said. I blushed and told him he looked handsome too. Both weddings were fun. My mom and dad were invited to the second wedding at the Ramada Hotel, so we sat with them and a few of my friends. We had so much fun dancing the night away. Near the end of the evening, I hinted that it would have been so much more convenient to have a hotel room instead of driving home. A few minutes later, Mick disappeared. When he returned he told me to check his jacket pocket. It was a hotel room key. "Perfect," I thought and smiled. Needless to say, we shared more than a goodnight kiss that night.

Mick and I got some breakfast the next morning and talked about the evening and our relationship. We were both on the same page. It was great. He dropped me off, and I told him to phone me when he got back to Langenburg. My parents didn't ask where I spent the night and obviously I didn't share either, but my mom did say she noticed how much fun I was having at the wedding. Mick and I chatted that evening for hours. I felt happy, genuinely happy.

When I got off the phone that night I remember thinking, "What would Mick think and do if he knew what I really was? Who would want to get involved with a girl that has serious emotional problems?" I portrayed a bubbly and friendly image in public, but I was something completely different on the inside; insecure and fragile. Without a doubt, I wore a mask to hide my emotional insecurities and mental health problems from others. I knew I had to tell Mick a bit about what I was doing to myself, but that was a scary thought for me. I was sure he would run the other way.

For the next few weeks, we continued talking on the phone. I was picking up more nursing shifts, and he was busy teaching and coaching volleyball on the weekends. His friend's wedding date in Langenburg was nearing. I made plans to take the bus to Yorkton, since I didn't have a vehicle. I decided to wait and see how the weekend went after meeting his friends and then maybe I would tell him more bulimia issues.

Mick picked me up in Yorkton on the Thursday night, and we drove to his place in Langenburg. His roommates were really nice. The wedding rehearsal was on Friday evening, and I got to meet the couple getting married. They were very friendly people, and I could see right away why Mick was buddies with the groom. The wedding ceremony was beautiful. I hung out most of the day with Mick's roommates because he was in the wedding party. The dance was a blast; Mick and I enjoyed dancing the night away. Small town weddings were awesome and I think I was falling for this small town boy.

I returned to Regina thinking about my dilemma of whether, or how, I should tell Mick about my "lifestyle". After a few evenings of chatting on the phone, I finally worked up the courage to tell him about my destructive habit. When I did, it seemed like he really didn't know much about bulimia, or perhaps he did and was just so shocked that he didn't know what to say. Mick mentioned, that he saw on television once, that celebrities and fashion models can sometimes struggle with eating disorders. That seemed to be the extent of his understanding of bulimia. I tried explaining with a bit more detail, of what I did, but I still downplayed the problem. I told Mick that I planned to stop practising the behavior very soon. After chatting for a while longer, he told me that he really cared about me. He even joked, "You're gonna have to do better than that to scare me off. Just let me know how I can help and I will be there for you."

I appreciated his words, but I can assure you, that Mick had no idea what he was getting himself into by dating me. I felt horrible and scared. I finally found a guy that was so different than all the other guys I've dated, and I was probably going to find a way to blow it. Actually, I didn't even have to try too hard, as my eating disorder was enough to hijack any relationship. I hoped not, because I felt like I could be myself around Mick. I could finally take off my mask. I didn't have to pretend to be something or someone I wasn't when I was with him. I felt a closeness and something genuine, so I prayed that my illness wouldn't derail this relationship. I knew in my heart, right then and there, that I wanted to spend the rest of my life with Mick.

GETTING BETTER FOR WHO ... THEM OR ME?

Months went by, and I continued working on the psychiatric unit. I was still getting called in at all hours of the night to the hospital, especially when a psych nurse was required for the constant observation of a new admission. Even though many of these new admissions demonstrated some pretty intense behaviors, I was never scared to pick up a shift. It didn't matter if I sat with a male or female. I was just happy to be involved in the first part of their treatment. On one occasion, I was called in at about 2:00 a.m. When I arrived to the emergency department the patient was sleeping. I relieved the E.R. nurse and sat down in the room. The patient was under his blanket but seemed to be a fairly big guy. Three hours went by before he woke up fairly agitated. I put down my magazine and said hello. He said, "Hi," and that he wanted to go out for a cigarette. He slipped out of his hospital bed and reached for his shoes. He was wearing a hospital gown and his jeans. After considering his request for a few seconds, I told him that I would have to go with him. As he stood up I realized that he was a big man, probably six feet, four inches tall and two hundred fifty pounds. He was still pretty irritated, but I was used to that type of behavior. I certainly wasn't going to get into a battle with him over a cigarette. We walked past the nurses' station, when one of the nurses asked me if she should call security. I told her not to bother as we were just going out for a smoke. I could tell she thought I was crazy to go outside with him by myself. As we passed through the exit doors, I laid down the ground rules. I lit up a smoke with him and said, "If you are thinking about running, I won't be chasing after you because I won't be able to stop you anyways. But then I will have to phone the police because you are a certified patient. When the police find you they will bring you right back to the hospital. I'm just guessing, but it probably won't be a very pleasant experience." He looked at me and replied, "Yeah, no worries, I get it, I just need a smoke, and we will go back in." We then started having a regular conversation. He was actually a nice guy who had some serious mental health problems. He wasn't a bad guy, he just needed some help ... just like me.

Bulimia was a big part of "me", much like the mental illnesses that controlled the lives of the patients I counselled in the psychiatric unit. Until now, I had no plans of stopping my bulimic habits because I didn't think I had any real reason to stop. Honestly, I still looked forward to my binges. It was usually pretty easy to get away with binging and purging because both of my parents were still working full time. I woke up every morning thinking about the food I would devour. I got an all too familiar thrill every time I went binge shopping. It was an exhilarating mission. Cakes, cookies, ice cream – I could hardly wait to get them home and begin stuffing my face. Occasionally, it was a challenge to bring the food into the house if someone was home, but otherwise it was smooth sailing. If someone was home, I would leave the food in the vehicle and run out later to sneak it in. I hung out in my room with my food and then called a friend. I always picked up my phone. I needed someone to talk to while I ate. I'm not sure if this distracted my attention away from what I was doing to myself or what, but I just felt more comfortable practising my behavior while I was chatting to a friend. Maybe if I had a television in my room that would have been a good enough too? On average, a grocery bag full of desserts would be about three trips to the bathroom. With my parents either downstairs or also talking on their phone, I was usually able to throw up without any concerns of someone hearing me. Occasionally, my mom knocked on the door asking if everything was okay; I always said yes. I would go through the same cycle each time. A rush and high of emotion surged through me as I gobbled up the food and then overwhelming feelings of guilt flooded in until I got the food out of me. As I began vomiting, I would slowly start to feel better. It was very important that I got everything out of my stomach by the time I was done my binge. Yellow juices from my stomach were a common sight in the toilet. My weight was about one hundred and twenty-five pounds, maybe one hundred thirty. I definitely wasn't losing weight by practising this behaviour, but as long as I didn't gain weight, I was okay with it.

Mick and I continued to talk almost every night. We were able to see each other about every second or third weekend. He never asked me too much about my bulimia. It was probably due to the fact that I kept my portions small when we were together so there were no warning signs for him. Plus, I had downplayed it and told him that I was going to put a stop to it soon. I was a textbook closet-eater who kept my secret by binging mostly in my bedroom. There was one bright side, since I had a phone in my bedroom, it gave me plenty of time to chat with Mick. We talked about everything (except my bulimia) and really got to know each other. There was always laughter in our conversations, and I really enjoyed that time with him even if it was just on the phone.

Mick and I had been dating about eight months. We began discussing a long-term future together. Mick applied for teaching positions in Regina and was short-listed for a job, so I was excited that he may be moving to Regina next fall. However, a couple days later he called to say that he had just been offered a temporary job as vice-principal of Langenburg High School. He didn't know what to do. I told Mick that he couldn't pass up an administration job, but we knew there was also some risk in passing up the Regina opportunity. Since the VP job was only a temporary position, he would have to interview again in a few months for a permanent contract if he enjoyed the new challenge.

Mick accepted the administrative position. I was very excited for him and couldn't wait to see him to celebrate as we were going to Watrous for the May long weekend. My sister Tammy lived there. On the way to Watrous, we envisioned our future together. I had done a four-month practicum at the Mental Health unit in Yorkton during my training, so I told Mick that maybe I should phone the director and see if there were any jobs available. As soon as the words came out of my mouth I remember thinking, "Wow. I could actually be moving to Langenburg." We both hoped things would work out. Our weekend in Watrous was great. Mick was a hit with my extended family, and they really welcomed him in with open arms.

When the weekend came to an end, I told Mick that I would phone Yorkton the next day. It turned out that there was a casual position at the Pine Unit. Holy cow, did that ever scare me. Was I once again trying to run away from my eating disorder? Could I handle all that change? I talked with my mom and dad that night. This move was much different than my Florida fiasco. My parents knew Mick pretty well by now and liked him, and the way he treated me. I think it was about a month later when I found myself in Langenburg with Mick and his two roommates. I started my orientation at the hospital a few days later. Yorkton was about a forty-five minute drive from Langenburg. I told myself that this would be a new beginning, which meant that I would stop throwing up. It didn't last. With Mick and his roommates all working, I had the place to myself the first few days I stayed there. No matter how hard I tried, I just couldn't stop binging and purging. I take that last statement back. I wasn't trying too hard or probably more accurately, not at all.

During the first couple weeks, the health district offered me a hotel room when I was scheduled for a night shift. It was part of the incentive package to get me to work in Yorkton. I stayed at the hotel a couple nights, however I actually phoned in sick on those evenings. Instead, since I was alone, I ran to the grocery store and loaded up on junk food. It was great. I had this whole room to myself and a ton of binge food. There was no one there to bother me during my raven-ous feasts. I sort of felt guilty that I didn't go to work, but I got over it pretty quickly. In reality, I was ill, but perhaps more mentally than physically. On my second day in the Yorkton hotel I went to the con-venience store to stock up. I had my bags of junk food and was walking back to the hotel, when I noticed a car in the parking lot that looked like Mick's. He had come to surprise me. I think my heart stopped beating but somehow I just kept on walking past the car. I threw the bags of groceries into a trash bin that was fortunately nearby and circled back to the hotel. I hoped to god that Mick didn't see me. How would I ever explain all that food? He knew I had a problem, but he definitely did not know how serious it was. Actually, I can't even call it a problem; it was my life. That was the first close call I had with him. I got to the elevator and Mick was there. I acted surprised to see him and gave him a big hug. I explained that I had phoned in sick, but we could still stay in the hotel overnight. I was so glad that he didn't see me in the parking lot ... that would have been a devastating start to my new beginning.

A few weeks later Mick and I started looking for a house in Langenburg as it was pretty crowded in the duplex with his roommates. We found a beautiful old character home. The price was right and next thing I knew we bought the house. It all seemed so surreal. Could it be that things would work out for me? Things were definitely coming together, yet I still was binging and purging every time I got a chance. Practising my behavior was going to be a trickier undertaking now that I was living in a small town, as it seemed like everybody knew what everyone else was doing. I was getting more shifts on the Psychiatric Unit in Yorkton, and I was enjoying my work. Sometimes after a shift, I would stock up on chocolate bars at the gas station. I would eat while driving back to Langenburg with the radio blasting, just in my own world. Then I would stop at the next gas station that came up and use their bathroom to puke it all out. Driving and eating was something I did often. It reduced my chances of getting caught. Thank God all the toilets in the gas stations worked. I kept up this routine for the next few months, but otherwise things were great. Our new character home was looking beautiful. We bought new furniture, painted, and were settling in nicely. We even bought a puppy named Jazzie together. We were very happy.

GOING TO THE CHAPEL AND I'M GOING TO GET MARRIED!

It was September 17, 2000, and it was Mick's birthday. We went to Regina to visit my parents. We had just finished supper when my mom came around the corner with a cake for Mick. We sang happy birthday to him and my dad prompted Mick to make a wish before blowing out the candles. Mick closed his eyes for what seemed like forever ... we all waited, and waited, wondering what he was wishing for that took so long. Finally, he opened his eyes and blew out the candles. My mom proceeded to grab the cake to cut it up, but she was interrupted by Mick kneeling down on one knee. I had no idea what he was doing. Then he looked up at me, pulled out an engagement ring and said, "With your family present, and with their permission, I would like to ask you something ... will you marry me?" I don't know who said yes first, me or my mom! I gave Mick a big hug and kiss and then put on the ring. It was absolutely beautiful. I found out later he had the ring custom-made by a jeweller. I was so happy. How much better could my life get!

About a month later, we went to Calgary so I could meet Mick's mom and dad. They were very friendly and excited for us. I got introduced to East Indian food. It was a bit spicy, but delicious. I was careful not to eat too much so that I didn't feel the need to purge. I really enjoyed getting to know his parents. They had moved from India to Canada in 1965. I met Mick's siblings while we were there too. They were all excited about our engagement. We discussed having dual ceremonies. An Indian ceremony at the temple back in Regina, as well as a Catholic service at my parent's church. It would bring two very different cultures together for a few days in order to celebrate our union. I was getting very excited about our big day.

When we got back to Langenburg I kept myself busy with wedding plans, but my eating disorder continued to control me. Funny how that works; the thing you think you have control over is actually the thing that's controlling you. Being bulimic was something that I did without consciously thinking about it. I can't exactly remember the first time that Mick "caught me", but gradually he was becoming more aware that my eating disorder may be more significant than he first thought. I began lying to him in order to keep him in the dark, but I could not sneak into the bathroom and throw up anymore when he was home. I tried to keep my binges to a minimum, but that wasn't working. I had to make the best of my time alone when Mick was at work. On a positive note though, I did start seeing a private counsellor through work. I remember my first session. I was so scared. How could I stop doing this when I didn't really want to? I said I wanted to stop, but that was just another lie.

I remember a really embarrassing incident that involved a big bag of chocolate-covered almonds. I was at home alone, so I decided to "snack" on them while I talked on the phone. Our puppy, Jazzie, started barking at me, so I threw her some without thinking or realizing that they could be harmful to her. I ate the whole bag while I chatted with my friend, minus the five that I threw to Jazzie. After purging, I went to the store and bought some more to replace the bag I ate. I was definitely good at covering my tracks, or so I thought. That night, while we were sleeping, Mick and I got awakened to Jazzie gagging. Mick jumped out of bed and turned on the light. Jazzie had vomited a bunch of small round objects. Looking puzzled, Mick picked one up and said, "These look like almonds, how did she get into those?" I felt my anxiety rise, but I knew I couldn't lie about it. I admitted to Mick that I had mistakenly tossed some of the chocolate treats to Jazzie. I can't remember what Mick said, but I know he was upset and frustrated as he figured out the scenario pretty quickly. When I think about that memory now, I can't believe that I was so focused on my binging that I almost hurt my puppy. That is just one of many disturbed events from the past that I can finally talk about. Please forgive me, Jazzie.

SEEKING SOME REAL HELP

Milden, Saskatchewan – population not even two hundred. This was the place where my healing journey began. It was January, 2001 when I found out about this disordered eating intervention facility at work. I discussed the program with Mick and my mental health counsellor. I made a call, and they sent me some information and registration forms. This was a very difficult time in my life. Mick and I had our wedding quickly approaching, and I wasn't doing any better. I can't speak for Mick, but I knew he didn't know what to do anymore. We both needed support to help me get me over this destructive disease.

My mom and Mick drove me to the BridgePoint Center For Eating Disorders which was a few hours from Regina. We arrived, and my anxiety was through the roof despite being prescribed Paxil for depression-anxiety-bulimia. I gave Mick and my mom a big hug and cried my eyes out as I would be there for three weeks.

I was greeted by some wonderful staff and taken to my room. I noticed there were two beds. I turned around and saw a girl ... her name was Debbie. It was a bit odd at first because we both really wanted a room to ourselves. We started chatting and shared our reservations about being at BridgePoint. Surprisingly, after a few minutes, I couldn't believe how comfortable I felt talking with her. We would later become soulmate friends.

Day 1 - The room was filled with thirteen girls. We all sat on the floor looking at each other. I felt a strange sense of belonging to this group of girls. Eating disorders was something that we had in common. We went around the room introducing ourselves. People shared their stories about what brought them there. As it got closer to my turn to speak, I could feel my anxiety escalating. "My name is Andrea Gilbert, and I am a Psychiatric Nurse. I am engaged to be married. My fiancé Mick is wonderful. I have been a bulimic for about thirteen years now. I have great parents, two sisters, and a brother.

They are all very supportive. As I was listening to all of you speak, I felt guilty because many of you don't have that same support system. Anyways, I am going to try to gain some self-awareness and maybe even learn how to stop throwing up."

As I put my head down on the pillow that night, I couldn't help but reflect on our sharing circle that evening. Almost every girl confided that they had been sexually abused as a child or adolescent. I felt so sorry for them. Maybe I didn't deserve to be here. My life was good, so I wondered why I had this disorder.

Day 2 - The next morning I woke up and had breakfast, which consisted of an apple and coffee. We met for our morning group and everyone was asked to do a "check-in". When a "check-in" was requested of you it meant that you were being asked to honestly express how you were feeling in that moment. It soon became common that most of the girls would start out saying they felt "fine", but soon had tears rolling down their cheeks, including myself. I knew I wasn't "mentally or emotionally okay" either, and I desperately wanted some magical potion to fix me, so that I could just go home to live happily ever after.

Attending an eating disorder clinic didn't mean that we just sat around talking about our feelings until we cried. We all needed to sign up for kitchen duties. We all took turns preparing meals and cleaning up. The kitchen was huge and full of all sorts of foods, some "good" and some "bad". At first I couldn't understand why we were allowed to be surrounded by the "bad" food. By "bad" foods I usually mean desserts, although sometimes that didn't matter to me. Often, I would eat just about anything … quantity over quality. I usually just ate a lot, and when I did … it didn't stay down.

After my first two days there, I was exhausted. I had an emotional cry in the afternoon group session. Our groups didn't focus on the food, because after all, it wasn't about the food. I get that now, but didn't back then. How could it *not* be about the food? Most of our time was spent on developing a strong sense of self-awareness. I remember one of the counsellors telling me that on my healing journey the *last* thing that would go away would be the behavior itself. "Wait a second," I thought, "Didn't I come here to learn how to stop throwing up?" I did, but I learned it definitely wouldn't stop overnight.

Day 3 - I was starting to adjust to my new routine. As far as eating, I decided to use my willpower and keep down anything I ate. This mostly consisted of veggies, fruit, and whole wheat bread. When it came to eating my thinking was definitely in an all or nothing state. My roommate and I were getting to know each other quite well and even having a few good laughs. I talked to Mick a few times. "Are you feeling any better yet?" he asked. "Well, I'm learning a lot about myself," I said. I wished it was that easy to quit binging and purging.

One of the amazing facilitators at BridgePoint was a non-practicing cocaine addict. I remember wondering what the heck he would know about eating disorders. It turned out that all addictions and addicts have many similarities. The facilitator spoke about the "Four A's of Recovery": Awareness, Acknowledgement, Acceptance, and Action. Learning about these four steps turned out to be quite an instrumental and an eye-opening moment. Many of the participants at BridgePoint, including myself, often became stuck between the phases of Acknowledgement and Acceptance. Let me explain this. Although we were *aware* that we all had a "food problem" and that we had *acknowledged* this by coming to BridgePoint, it still didn't mean that we had truly *accepted* the seriousness of our illness. By simply attending a disordered eating clinic also didn't mean that we had yet taken any routine *action* to change our daily and self-destructive habits. However, without question, attending BridgePoint was a significant beginning in our healing continuum, as it instilled hope that a healthier life was possible.

One of our group activities was called Creative Expressions. We were asked to bring a sketchbook with us to this session. We'd close our eyes and try to tune in to our physical feelings. We were then given pastels to draw with. I didn't realize the purpose of this activity as I was more concerned about making a pretty picture than actually letting my hands just color or draw how I felt at that moment. We then each had an opportunity to explain our picture. I didn't know what to say about this swirl of colors in front of me, so that's what I said. The counsellor asked me why, and I explained the fear I had inside about not making a nice picture. "Then that's exactly what it is," she said. "Ah-ha," I thought, "that actually makes sense." My whole life I was more concerned about what others thought of me, or trying so hard to impress others, instead of just being myself. For some reason, approval from others seemed to be number one on my list of needs. I sometimes find it awkward to talk about my life back then, especially when I reflect on my mental health … but I wouldn't change a thing, as it has all brought me to where I am today.

The days continued to roll on at BridgePoint and things seemed to be going well. By going well, I mean that at least I was still there, and I didn't run away and give up. I didn't throw up once and that made me believe that I was doing well. I had some pretty intense moments and there were many tears. I watched other girls binge and purge over the entire three week program. I felt sorry for them because I felt like I was doing so much better than them. Mick and my family also came up for the family and friends weekend. I really appreciated their support, and I had to get better *for them*.

HERE WE GO AGAIN

I arrived back home with a whole new outlook on life. I hadn't binged and purged for three weeks, and I didn't want to blow it. That attitude lasted for about four days. The anxiety of not being able to eat what I wanted got to me. I just wanted one cookie, so I had one and then the whole bag. It was like a powerful drug that just took over my mind. Once I stuffed myself, I felt full of shame and guilt. As fast as I gobbled down the food, I wanted it out even quicker. A big sigh of relief followed when I flushed the toilet. That physical feeling of relief didn't last long. I once again had attempted to overcome this abnormal and destructive behavior but failed. The "same old, same old" Andrea was back. I felt so defeated that I didn't think I was ever going to be able to stop. Occasionally, these moments of reality would smack me in the face. Any reflection on my destructive habits would not only fill me with guilt, but also scare the hell out of me ... would I ever be able to quit?

On the other hand, I could escape reality when I binged and purged. It helped me regain a sense of control ... as food was the one thing that I felt was within my grasp to control. In retrospect, these feelings of control were most definitely misleading, as my self-harming addiction was in control of my life. I know the dichotomy sounds strange, but I felt a very self-reassuring "high" when I binged. Miraculously, I was able to "survive" in this state of tug-of-war turmoil for many years. Not only was I able to give medication at work without any error, but I was often praised for my professional connection and care for our psychiatric patients and special care home residents. Somehow, I was always emotional and cognitively present for people in my care. Maybe taking care of others made me forget about my own issues.

So, I tried to remind myself that not all was bad. There were several positive things happening in my life at this time. I would soon be marrying the man of my dreams. As a couple, we owned and remodelled a beautiful character home in Langenburg. In addition, I was meeting new people and developing new friendships. Regardless of all this, I still needed my self-harming addiction ... it trumped everything else.

DREAM WEDDING(S)!

July 14, 2001 ... one year after my grandpa had passed away. I arrived at the temple at 8:00 a.m. dressed beautifully in my Indian wedding dress. My makeup was flawless, and my smile was bright. I was so happy that this day was finally here. The ceremony was such a special experience. I was thrilled because I knew that having this cultural ceremony meant so much to Mick's parents. Shortly after, I changed into my second wedding dress for the Catholic wedding ceremony and, surprisingly, I actually liked what I saw in the mirror. Maybe it was because I was filled with so much excitement and joy that I was able to overlook my usual body image concerns. My mom and dad walked me down the aisle and "gave me away". The service was so beautiful. We had our reception at a big hall in Regina. There was around five hundred people in attendance, and the evening couldn't have been more perfect. I felt like the luckiest person on earth. I never once thought about binging the entire day. Maybe it was because I knew I couldn't get away with it? Too many people had their eyes on me.

The next day was the gift opening at my parents' house. My family did a wonderful job of decorating, and there was tons of food. One of our gifts was a honeymoon trip leaving in one week. Mick was in on the surprise with his buddy. We were going to St. Maarten, Virgin Islands! I was so excited and wanted these next few weeks to last forever. We went back to Langenburg for a few days with all of our gifts from the wedding. My mom and dad, my brother, his girlfriend, Mick's parents, and my aunt and uncle from Australia all came back with us to continue the celebration. I was so touched that everyone could come out to Langenburg. We had a few friends over for the evening and had a barbeque. My dad even brought fireworks and asked the mayor for permission to shoot them off that evening. It was a great party. I was so happy and thanked God for the blessings in my life.

We returned to Regina a few days later. We saw my Australian uncle and aunt off at the airport. I was still so touched that they flew all that way for my wedding. Our flight left for St. Maarten the next day. It was such a beautiful island. I love the ocean and always have. Watching the sunrise on the beach with a coffee was amazing. There is something so mesmerizing about the tide. I felt the strength of the waves and respected the power they possessed. Between the sun and the waves, I was in heaven. The whole week that we were there, using my willpower, I was able to eat moderate amounts of food and not feel the urge to throw up. How could this be a problem if I was able to control it? I was very proud of myself. Little did I know at the time, but this new "found" control was due to my "all-or-nothing" thinking rather than my ability to self-regulate. It felt like self-control, but I was restricting my diet once again … and that wasn't a good option for me either. Instead, the dieting just kick-started another vicious cycle of bulimia that would continue to consume my life.

THE HONEYMOON ENDS

Once we arrived back in Langenburg not only did the honeymoon come to an end, so did my willpower. I had gone for over two weeks without throwing up, but as soon as I got the chance to binge I embraced the opportunity. My thoughts shifted back to food, just like that. The stress involved in planning the binges was overwhelming. I was constantly thinking of my next binge and how to be increasingly secretive about it. I couldn't buy all my food locally because we lived in a small town. It really worked out well when I had to work in Yorkton. I always ate lunch in the cafeteria and then threw up in my favorite toilet at the hospital (just like I had done in Regina for many years). Again, I would never eat an amount that people would question, as I wanted to portray the image of a healthy young lady to my colleagues. As I write these last few pages, I realize the repetitiveness in my story. It reminds me of the many failed attempts I experienced in my quest to rid myself of bulimia and reaffirms the cyclical nature of this disease.

Being alone (of course) was my favorite past time. It allowed me to prepare my feasts in peace, turn on the TV, and chow down. I would zone out, in a world of my own, with no one there to judge me. I looked forward to these times more than anything else. I could take off my mask and be myself, just me and my illness. I was in total control during these times, and that thrilled me. The sensation may have been similar to how a drug addict feels when they are hooked up to their drug of choice. The mind altering behavior was quite empowering.

Not surprisingly, this disordered behaviour was not only emotionally and physically taxing, but financially as well. Whether you need to buy cocaine, alcohol, or food, it all costs money. I had my job as a nurse, so that helped, but now that I was married I wasn't just spending my money. Now I was spending our money, Mick's paycheque as well, but that didn't slow me down. My addiction had cost me thousands of dollars over the years. I don't think I realized the strain this would put on our marriage, or maybe I did and I just didn't care. I'd also like to say that I felt bad or sorry about spending "our money" on my addiction, but I'm not certain that I did. I sure feel terrible about it now though.

I continued to be an "unnoticed" bulimic at work. Even though I had an addiction, I felt I had control over my behavior, so I could wear my mask at work and be an effective nurse. My weight was about one hundred and twenty pounds and I was five foot three inches, so I considered that pretty average-sized. After getting married, my life finally seemed to be working out just fine for me. I was able to juggle work and my disorder. I had a great husband, a good job, and an eating disorder that was all mine.

Like all the other times, this perfect scenario developed some glitches. It was getting more difficult to be sneaky around home and work. Sometimes I thought that it took more energy to binge and purge, than it did to work. I liked my job and was able to handle the difficult patients that were admitted to the psychiatric unit. However, I do recall a day when we had a very mentally ill patient. He was a large older man who had a history of major aggression. He was in his room with the psychiatrist. All of a sudden we heard the man yelling from the room and some banging noises. The nurse in charge immediately called the main hospital switchboard and reported what was going on. A "code white" was announced over the intercom. Code white translates basically to violent patient. Next thing I knew the unit was being flooded with psychiatrists, more nurses, and security. They lined up in the hallway outside of the patient's room. I was still at the desk with another nurse. One of the nurses came running out of the room and told us that doctor orders were to give the patient a sedative by injection. I almost stopped breathing instantly, because I was the medication nurse that day, and that meant I would have to give the injection.

The other nurse looked at me and said, "Come on, Andrea. You need to get the medication drawn up right now." I remember looking down the hallway and seeing the twenty or more professionals looking at the desk. I grabbed the antipsychotic medication vial, and the nurse handed me a needle and syringe. My hands were shaking so much that my colleague offered to draw the medication into the syringe. "Can you just give him the injection for me?" I asked. Her response was something I will never forget. "Andrea, I probably could do it for you, but how does that help you? I know you are nervous, but all of us are too. Just focus on giving him the needle and pretend no one else is there. I know you can do it."

Seconds later, needle in hand, I made my way to his room. When I got there the man was sitting on the bed beside his doctor. There were three other nurses in the room as well. "Hello, Mr. Edwards. My name is Andrea, and I'm going to give you a little something to help calm you down." I waited for his response, holding the needle in front of him. "Okay, but I want it given in my arm," he said. "Great",

I thought. We had put a two inch needle on the syringe because we usually give it in the gluteus muscle, also known as the butt. I knew that I didn't have time to mess around with changing the needle. "Just insert it in half way," one of my co-workers said. I don't know where my burst of confidence came from, but the next thing I knew I was pulling the empty syringe out of his arm. "I barely felt that," the man said. I thanked him for his cooperation and left the room. Back at the desk, when everyone that rushed to the unit was gone, Nurse Sharon told me I did great. I thanked her for helping me, by not helping me. I think you know what I mean.

Back at home, when Mick and I were on days off together, I tried very hard to control my urges. I didn't want to lie to him and yet I did. We would enjoy a breakfast together, and I would wait for him to go into the shower. I would run downstairs and throw up in the toilet. In the moment, when this would go on, I didn't think about anything else. I was obviously still not ready to give up the behavior.

By now, I also made many good friends in Langenburg. I didn't tell them about my eating disorder though and I doubt they suspected bulimia based on what they saw me eat. For the most part, I ate healthy foods in front of others. Some of my friends may have thought I was a bit thin, but overall they probably saw an "average girl" that liked talking and laughing. In reality, I was very different from what I displayed publicly.

I continued going to therapy sessions in Yorkton. My therapist was not only compassionate, but also a good listener. I felt comfortable talking to him about my secretive lifestyle. I always felt so determined right after a therapy session, hoping this would be the day that I quit my self-harming behaviours.

One day, Mick unexpectedly came home early from work. My heart was racing when I heard the door open. I shoved whatever sweets I had into the kitchen cupboard. Hopefully there was no chocolate on my face or puke left in the toilet. Unfortunately for me, there was remains of vomit in the toilet, and he saw it. He got mad, and we had an argument about it. I tried to tell him that I was getting better and that I was reducing the amount of binges. Not totally true, so I didn't blame him at all for being upset. He had been so supportive up until now, but he didn't know how to help anymore. These incidents were becoming a regular occurrence in our marriage, so I wondered how Mick was coping.

As a result, I decided I needed to go back to the BridgePoint Center For Eating Disorders a second time. I had kept in contact with some of the staff and my roommate from the first visit. Debbie decided to give BridgePoint another try as well. Mick agreed with my decision. I'm sure he was praying that this second retreat would help me more than the first one.

BRIDGEPOINT 2.0

Fall 2001 – Debbie and I drove to Milden together. We had so much in common that we became very good friends. She even attended my wedding. We later recalled that we had previously worked a few casual shifts together at the Regina psychiatric unit before meeting at BridgePoint. Another strange coincidence. Our connection was very unique, and I am so glad we became such close friends. It's funny what can bring people together.

Luckily, once again Debbie and I were roommates. Many of the girls that attended BridgePoint on my first visit were there again. The environment had a familiar feel, except that some of the facilitators were different. When we arrived, I felt like a failure because I had to come back a second time. Why couldn't I just be stronger and stop this ridiculous habit? I put those thoughts aside and committed to being engaged in the program. Our groups were a continuation of the work we did in the first module and we always had the daily "check-ins". We had a morning check-in, another after lunch, and then a final one in the evening. "I feel like I'm going to explode," some girls would say right after eating a meal. I guess that's what stuffing not only your mouth, but also your feelings felt like. Many of us felt a defeated sense of guilt after eating. Then the guilt created an overwhelming need to throw up. Purging not only the food out, but more importantly those "stuffed feelings" as well. I usually didn't get those "I'm about to explode feelings" while I was at BridgePoint because I restricted my diet. Was it a sign of self-control and healing this time? Probably not. It didn't work last time, so why would it work on this visit? This time I decided that I really wanted to focus on my inner-self and figure out the root of my problems. I also wanted to do some exercising to get into better shape. Conveniently, there was an exercise and yoga room at BridgePoint.

One group session we participated in focused on relaxation techniques. This included deep breathing exercises. A participant volunteered for the demonstration. She was told to lie down on the floor, and the instructor asked her to relax and imagine herself feeling as light as a feather. It was very hypnotic. We were all quiet and watched intently. I soon felt myself getting very lightheaded. After that things got quite hazy, but I remember running out of the room and feeling like I couldn't breathe.

One of the staff came after me, along with my friend Deb. I sat down on a chair and tried to focus on what they were telling me to do. "Take slow deep breaths Andrea, you're okay, we are right here." I think I may have lost consciousness briefly because I felt all tingly and everything went black. My friend Deb had her arm around me the entire time. I started rocking in her arms, which grounded me. My breathing normalized, and I started feeling present again. I had never experienced anything like that before. The staff reassured me that I was physically okay and that I experienced a "flashback". What the hell is up with that? I didn't remember any details from the "flashback", but it certainly created some overwhelming emotions. The only thing

I could recall was that I was really frightened and felt like I was going to pass out.

Later on that same day we had our evening tea-time. We all sat in a circle on the floor with the lights dimmed and the candles lit. I really enjoyed these evenings. We had tea-time on Fridays, so I got to participate in three sessions in my previous visit to BridgePoint. This was our first session on this visit. We each got a turn to talk about whatever we wanted from our past, good or bad. I was feeling relaxed as I stared into the flames of the burning candles. I was barely listening to people share their feelings. I again felt like I was in some sort of trance. When it was my turn to speak, nothing came out of my mouth. I could feel tears running down my face. My friend Debbie was beside me, and she once again wrapped her arms around me. I couldn't explain why I was crying. I skipped my turn so others could continue sharing. The staff asked me afterwards how I was feeling. I didn't have the words to explain. I just knew I was exhausted.

I fell asleep shortly after slipping into my bed. As usual, I had the soothing music of Andrea Bocelli playing to relax my body and bring some peacefulness to my mind. My sleep, however, was often filled with strange dreams. That evening I dreamt of my sister Kim. She and I were at our babysitter's house. We were quite young in the dream. The dream began with us walking through a big old house. The only other person in my dream is our babysitter. Kim and I walk up to his bedroom door and open it. He is standing in his room wearing a blue robe. We stand in front of him as he takes off his robe. He is completely naked and smiles at us. He asks us to touch him.

Then next morning I woke up feeling like I hadn't slept a wink. My mind was thinking about that blue robe. I thought, "What a totally bizarre dream!" I didn't want to over analyze it because I often had weird dreams, so maybe this was just one more. I didn't know it at the time, but in more recent years when I shared my "babysitter dream" with Kim, she hesitantly confided that it wasn't "just a dream". She told me that it was a memory.

The remainder of my two weeks at BridgePoint was overflowing with emotion. I continued to learn more about myself. I became really aware of how much of a people-pleaser I was. I worried about what people thought of me more than I worried about what I thought of myself. Exploring your inner being was emotionally draining. I don't think any of the participants at BridgePoint really liked "looking in the mirror". Or at least, I know I didn't. My eating patterns were the same as my first go around, I was still restricting myself and thinking I was doing well … go figure!

We still had two days left before we were supposed to go home. Deb and I decided that we were ready to go home, like today … like right now. The staff encouraged us to stay until the program was completed, but we had already made up our minds. We felt complete. And so we left. We truly felt like we didn't need any more daily check-ins and support groups.

SISTERS' CONNECTION

Since BridgePoint is in southwest Saskatchewan, on my way back to Langenburg I spent a few days at my parents' house before heading back home. My sister Kim was living there at the time, so I wanted to stop in and visit her as well. Kim had been diagnosed with Multiple Sclerosis in her early twenties, so she was battling through her own medical issues. Kim and I were in the garage having a smoke, and I don't know what made me think of it, but I started telling her about a few of my bizarre dreams. I always felt like I was falling in my dreams. Some of the dreams woke me up in a panicky sweat. Often I remember trying to scream, but nothing seemed to come out of my mouth. I would try to get someone's attention, but my cries for help were muffled so nobody heard me. Kim shared that day that she too had some very similar dreams over the years.

I must be careful how I share this next thought out of respect for my sister. As we began to share more with each other over the years, I realized that Kim had been exposed to some awful experiences in her childhood. Experiences that no child should ever have to deal with. My sister has confided in me, and I have promised not to repeat the details, but I do feel bad for her as she has had a very tough life so far. Not only did MS kick the shit out of her for many years, which may have resulted in her boyfriend of almost nine years breaking up with her, but she also shared something that added even more devastation to her life story. It definitely wasn't fair what happened to her. I wanted to tell my parents so badly, but I had to respect my sister's wishes. As sisters, we will be there for each other no matter what the future brings our way.

DENTAL NIGHTMARE

Back to Langenburg I went. How was I doing physically? Well, let's start with my teeth. I hadn't been to the dentist for a few years as I was embarrassed by my teeth. I know my eating disorder had done significant damage. The four teeth at the front and top of my mouth were really starting to thin. The enamel was wearing off due to prolonged acid exposure during my purges. Did I really think there would be no consequences from this harmful addiction? Actually, no. I honestly never thought about the harm I was doing to my body. It just didn't matter. The only thing that mattered was the high I got from binging and purging. This was just the way I chose to live my life and to me it usually seemed perfectly normal.

I finally convinced myself that I probably should make an appointment with the dentist for an examination and a cleaning. I remember driving to my appointment feeling nervous, scared, and extremely anxious. I knew that the dentist would figure out within minutes of looking into my mouth that I was a bulimic. The receptionist called my name. The moment of shame had arrived. I know many people don't like going to the dentist. That's pretty common. Patients are often either scared of the drill sounds or hate keeping their mouth open for an extended period of time, while others can't stand the smell of the dental office. For me, it was all of those things plus the fear of being exposed. I was ashamed that I would have to admit that I had an eating disorder. What would the dentist think of me? How could anyone feel sorry for someone that is deliberately wrecking their teeth and harming their body?

I entered the room and sat on the dentist chair. My heart was racing so fast that I must have looked nervous. The dentist introduced himself. My first impression was that he seemed empathetic and non-judgmental. That made me feel more comfortable. We discussed the specific teeth that were bothering me. There were a few. "Well, let's get that X-ray and we will go from there," the dentist said. While I was waiting for him to come back and discuss the X-ray findings, I decided that this time I would just come out and tell him about my issues. He was a smart guy and would figure it out anyways. His assistant came into the room and put my X-rays on the screen as this was before the digital X-ray era. The assistant and I engaged in some small talk until the dentist walked in. It was the moment of truth. I just blurted it out, "I'm bulimic." He stared at me for a few moments, and his assistant was quiet. Then the tears started to flow, and I was a mess. I tried to calm myself down and focus on where I was. This wasn't my counsellor's office or BridgePoint. This was the dental office. Fortunately, he was quite compassionate, even though I really don't think I deserved the empathy.

I was right. My front teeth were thinning and there was a chance that the tips could crack or chip in the near future. I also had several cavities and one tooth that would eventually need to be extracted. The dental plan was … one tooth at a time. I wasn't sure what my insurance coverage was or if we could afford the cost of all this work. Once again, my eating disorder was not only causing me health issues, but it was possibly going to be a financial strain on our marriage as well.

CAUGHT IN ANOTHER LIE

A couple weeks after the dental visit, Mick caught me in a humiliating lie. He had gone off to work that morning as usual. I was planning my day … meaning all the food I was going to eat. Let's see, first, I will start with about four pieces of toast smothered with butter, peanut butter, and jam. Then, of course, I will need to drink a big glass of milk. I always made sure to "drink plenty of fluids" between the mouthfuls of food. Without liquids, purging dry foods was a very difficult and often painful process. So, I guess this was my way of trying not to damage my esophagus … I know, it sounds ridiculous. Also, most "normal" human beings would be concerned about harming their teeth in any manner, especially after seeing the dentist, but not me. Next, a big bowl of cereal was on the menu. It really didn't matter what kind of cereal it was, but there were some foods that I absolutely preferred over others, like chocolate bars for breakfast. Why not? Technically, it wasn't breakfast if you didn't keep it down, right?

After gulping down the food, I went to the tap to get some water and nothing came out of the spout. I instantly felt my heart start to pound. For some reason the town water supply was off, which meant the toilet wouldn't flush either. I was over-stuffed with four pieces of toast, a bowl of cereal, and three chocolate bars. Yikes, I needed to get this bloated feeling out of me now! I quickly decided to use Plan B. This was something I had done before and most of the time things worked out just fine. I quickly grabbed a large Glad Ziploc bag and chugged back a bottle of water. I then bent over, held the bag open, and puked my guts out. What an instant sense of relief. Talk about a love-hate relationship with food. Okay, next step, what to do with this bag filled with puke? For now, I would seal it tight and put it in the garbage. Once the water came back on I could dump it in the toilet. I was good, Plan B seemed adequate. An instant later, to my shock, I heard the front door open. It scared the living shit out of me. It was Mick. He came home to get something he needed for work. My instinctive reaction was to grab the bagful of puke out of the garbage and run downstairs. I slid into the laundry room and hid the Ziploc bag full of warm vomit under a pile of clothes on the floor. Luckily I hadn't done laundry in a few days, so I opened the washing machine lid and threw in a few clothes. I figured it would be best if I pretended like I was doing the laundry … dah … impossible, the water supply was off!

Mick came downstairs, "Andrea, didn't you hear me come in?" he suspiciously asked, "And then I saw you running down the stairs, what's up?" Of course, I tried lying my way out of the predicament. I told Mick that I didn't hear him and that I must have been just heading downstairs to do laundry when he walked in the house. He gave me the most distraught look of disappointment that I will never forget. I then knew he didn't believe me. I was so flustered that I told him I had to go upstairs. I was terrified that he would find the evidence of my lies. But why would he go digging through a pile of dirty clothes though? Maybe I was overreacting and had nothing to worry about … wrong again.

The next thing I knew, Mick came storming upstairs and was holding the bag full of regurgitated food right in front of my face. My heart sank. "What the hell is this? I thought you said you weren't throwing up anymore!" he yelled. I felt frantic. I'm sure Mick felt like he had just caught me with another man. Without a doubt, he was probably disappointed in me and in our marriage. I knew he was upset, probably totally disgusted, and there was nothing I could say in my defense to make it better this time. The bag ended up in the sink. Mick said that he couldn't take the lies anymore and stormed out of the house for work. I spent the rest of the day on pins and needles wondering what was going to happen. Was our marriage over? Fortunately, although I'm not sure why, once the emotional tension subsided and we had a chance to talk, Mick decided to give me another chance to stop all the bullshit lies. I promised to get more help. I had to do something, otherwise I was sure that my marriage would be a very short one. I didn't want to have to choose between my husband and my eating disorder. I wanted them both. This attitude left many unanswered questions. How can someone continue to hurt themselves and the people they love? What was it going to take to cure myself? Even though I wasn't ready to give up in this fight yet, realistically I knew that I probably wouldn't figure out the answer to these questions for a very long time, or maybe never.

BRIDGEPOINT 3.0

Another Christmas came and went and so did the food. I don't think I need to go into the details as I'm sure you know how it went. This was the time of year when people make resolutions to begin the New Year with a positive attitude and a healthy lifestyle. My resolutions were too difficult to do on my own. I've had an eating disorder for almost fifteen years now. The human body sure can endure a lot of abuse. I guess that's what kept me going. I continued abusing my body and finding a way to get my fix, so it's not surprising that I found myself phoning BridgePoint to inquire if a bed was available in their the next module.

January 2002 – I was back at the BridgePoint Center For Eating Disorders once again. I hoped, like they say, that the third time's a charm! I sure as hell hoped so, as I knew my marriage depended on it. My friend Debbie didn't come with me this time. I met some new people and reconnected with some past participants. My parents knew I was going to BridgePoint, but I hadn't told them what happened at home with Mick.

In retrospect, this disease was so easy to slip into and is much easier to hide than other addictions. It's not like trying to get a hold of an illicit drug, food is everywhere. I also haven't met a bulimic who openly eats copious amounts of food in front of others or isn't discreet about their trips to the washroom. The behaviour would be public knowledge pretty quick without discretion. To be "successful" a bulimic needs to figure out how to manipulate the many variables in their life, especially the people they love.

I looked up the definition of being **manipulative** and here's what I found: *Influencing or attempting to influence the behavior or emotions of others for one's own purposes. Synonyms: scheming, calculating, cunning, crafty, shrewd, devious, sly, artful, disingenuous, and selfish.* There were even more uncomplimentary words listed, but those pretty much sum up exactly how I behaved. Not characteristics that I was really proud of or would like to pass on to my future kids. The ironic thing was that I really obsessed about what people thought of me and I needed to be liked. I do truly care about people. That's why I became a psychiatric nurse. I can totally relate to people who struggle with their mental health. Yet at the same time, this disease had such a strong hold over me that despite all my psychiatric knowledge and my work experience I still couldn't help myself but to manipulate situations to get my fix of food. I often lost my moral compass, especially when it came to my own health and my relationship with my husband. Unfortunately, it seemed like I was often choosing "it" over "me and him".

Maybe I could add *secretive* to that list of synonyms. When I look at the list of words I think, "Is this how I wanted to be viewed by others?" Of course not. That's where the word *secretive* comes in. Most people who know me would probably describe me as caring, funny, talkative, empathetic, and generous. That is the complete opposite of manipulative. It's puzzling how I was able to make all of these conflicting characteristics work in unison. It's almost amazing when I really think about it. However, I also know that it was very exhausting.

I drove myself to BridgePoint this time; I'm not sure if it was because I wanted to go on my own or if it was because my family was getting tired of, or used to, Andrea "going for help" again. It was about a five-hour trip. Once and for all, I really wanted to get rid of this disease. We wanted to have children, and I wasn't getting any younger. Upon arrival I spotted many familiar faces and some new ones too. We were all there to overcome our eating disorders: anorexia, bulimia, and obesity from overeating. So despite our unique and separate lives, we were all the same in many ways.

I got settled in my room, and we met for introductions. Since it was my third time there, I didn't feel as anxious. I knew that I was in a safe environment. "Hello, everyone. My name is Andrea Parmar and this is my third time at BridgePoint. I am a newlywed and have a wonderful husband. My parents are supportive too." There was that word supportive again. All it meant was that my family hadn't given up on me yet, as they couldn't do the difficult recovery work for me. "My parents live two hours from me, so they don't always know how I am really doing. My husband is getting quite frustrated and tired of my lies. He told me that he has a hard time trusting me. I mean, really, who wouldn't? I don't know how many more lies I can get away with. I want to have children soon. I'm here because I want to stop throwing up, but I'm scared I won't be able to do that. I don't even really know if I want to stop. Does that make sense?" Everyone nodded with agreement. "I feel like my eating disorder is a part of who I am and what would I be if I didn't have it. Yeah, I guess, once in a while I think about the physical damage I'm doing to myself, but I keep doing it anyways. I guess that's why it's an addiction." I could feel the tears building up inside of me, and I felt like a volcano that was ready to erupt, "I think that's all I want to say for now."

I listened to the rest of the group introductions. We all came from different places. We all looked different and our ages ranged from nineteen to sixty years old. When we spoke though, it was like we were identical twins. The stories of the daily struggles with food and the constant need to be in control seemed very familiar to all of us. We all thought we were controlling the food to get "our high", but in reality it couldn't be further from the truth. As a result of this denial, each and every one of us was "screwed up". Some struggled with an eating disorder for a few years and others for several decades. However, no matter how young or old, we all knew that we should be very thankful that our life paths had steered us towards BridgePoint. This "place" provided us with *hope*.

CAN I DO THIS? SHOULD I EVEN BOTHER?

As I reflect on the past decade, and as I type these words, there are many thoughts and feelings that flow through me. The whole point of journaling is to get your thoughts out on paper so that you can actually see them. When I first started this journal I was really excited and was typing just about every day. That lasted for about a week, maybe two. Like many things in my life, I enthusiastically started projects, but I often didn't finish them. This journal, this memoir, this book, or whatever you want to call it, is something that I can truly say I am doing, first and foremost, for myself. I know it's not written perfectly, and I'm okay with that. I have strived for perfection my whole life and I have beaten myself up for almost two decades because of it. So knowing that my writing is not perfect and being okay with that is a huge leap in personal self-worth for me. Being at peace with an imperfect recollection of my life struggles may just be another step in my healing.

Despite journaling my story, I recognize that I still have high expectations for myself and I still worry about what others think of me. Also, if I don't finish something, or don't reach a personal goal, it makes me feel like a failure … and if I'm a failure, who will like me? I'm afraid that is just how my brain works. I'm working at changing the "tapes that play in my head" because I know they negatively impact my self-concept. I also know it will take time to change my thinking as I've carried these self-criticizing thoughts in my head for many years. So yes, I still do feel like a failure sometimes and believe that I am the only person that feels this way. When I'm feeling more optimistic I realize that this is not true, but when I'm low, I do feel very alone in my head.

Occasionally, anxiety and panic attacks overwhelmed me. If you have never experienced a panic attack, you don't know what you're missing! It usually starts with a negative thought, or being in a situation that you think you can't handle. Almost instantly, a tingling and numbing sensation gushes over and paralyzes you. You often feel dizzy and have difficulty breathing. Believe me they are not fun. Over this past decade there were times when I began to feel anxious as I was journaling. The intent of journaling and the resulting feelings seemed to be an oxymoron. Reflecting upon the dark moments in my life were supposed to promote healing. Yet, at times, this reflection created new feelings of anxiety and emotional stress. I suppose it makes sense that these physiological reactions were triggered by unaddressed emotional baggage from the past. After the fact, I can now say that these anxiety-filled moments of reflection were key in progressing my healing. Being honest with myself, about the ugly truths of my past, was often a very difficult but necessary task.

WHY ME?

Once again, there were several new facilitators at BridgePoint on this third visit, however I presumed that many of the activities, experiences, and feelings would be the same as my previous two stays. For the most part, I was right, but there was one thing that was definitely different. *The difference was me.* Even though the same "speeches" were often being given by the staff, my reaction to them was different. I was no longer the same person. I was learning something new about myself on a daily basis. My main goal or question on this visit was to figure out why I was bulimic and what drove me to make these types of choices? I come from a good family, I have a fulfilling career, and now a wonderful husband. So why me?

I found myself regularly asking this question when things went wrong or when I felt sick. I don't think any human in the *right state of mind*, when given the choice whether to have something bad happen to them, would say, "Sure," and agree to the hardship. Do people choose to have cancer? Are people "okay" with getting into a life-changing car accident? No. People don't choose to be physically sick, critically injured, or mentally ill. So a question that really troubled me was … Did I have a choice? Did I choose this eating disorder? If not, what is driving me to continue this hurtful behavior? Or, if I do have a choice, why haven't I made a better one yet?

Maybe we don't always have a choice. My mother's mom didn't ask to be stricken with stage four cancer, at the age of twenty-nine, while being seven months pregnant. At the age of eleven, my mom didn't want to lose her mom and be thrust into new responsibilities with three younger siblings. So why do these bad things happen to us? How can they be fair? I didn't ask to get an eating disorder. I didn't plan on lying to my family and friends for all these years … but I have. Am I choosing to hurt people in my life, just so I can get my fix of food? I don't have the answers to all these questions yet, but I hope

I will soon, before something happens to my health, my marriage, or with my family that I cannot fix.

I don't intend for this journal, or this next passage, to be religious in any manner. That being said, I am Christian but I live more of a spiritual life than a religious one. The words of the Serenity Prayer truly resonate with me. A very dear friend and neighbor, the boys called her Grandma Terry even though she was of no blood relationship, gave me a bookmark as a gift once with these words on it:

"God grant me the serenity to accept the things I cannot change, courage to change the things I can, and the wisdom to know the difference."

Fast forward to today. After being alive for almost forty-five years, being a registered psychiatric nurse, having overcome bulimia, and finding the strength to resist the temptations of other addictions, the "Serenity Prayer" is the most simplistic, yet impactful advice that I have ever been given. The phrase just made complete sense to me the day I read it. Having the discipline to surrender to the things that I have no control over ... good or bad ... and then making the best decisions that I can in the situations where I do have some control, was another shift in mindset for me. I wish I had embraced this wisdom much earlier in life. I now realize that "we are who we are" because of our personal experiences and the choices we make along the way. This includes the scars, the pain, and the lessons we learn in our failures.

Over the many years of my recovery, I was eventually able to let go of the haunting question of "Why Me?" As I slowly learned more about myself, and about my mental illness, I was able to come to this conclusion ... Avoid getting stuck on these "why" questions. Trying to satisfy your relentless curiosity of your haunting past rarely supports a healthy recovery process. Actually, quite the contrary, there is a reasonable chance that it will instead exhaust you. Once I learned to "focus on today instead of yesterday" a heavy weight seemed to lift from my shoulders. With this shift in thinking, I was able to direct my energy in a more productive manner and soon noticed improvements in my mental health. The word "resilience" comes to mind when I think of dealing with past demons. So, instead of wallowing in past hardships, try to focus your energy on replacing the negative self-talk that swirls around in your mind with positive self-talk. This renewal and retraining of how you think will take every ounce of energy you have, so please don't continue to waste your energy on the "why me" questions like I did for many years.

Back to my days at BridgePoint … time seemed to be flying by very quickly this third time around. As far as my eating disorder, I restricted my intake (as usual) and stuck to eating the same safe foods. The facility's staff were amazing, and the group sessions helped gain more self-awareness about my personal and emotional "triggers". Obviously, Christmas was a big trigger for me. My mom was one of those ladies who would make enough food to feed an entire army. I experienced a variety of emotions around Christmas. I felt excited because I would get to eat all the Christmas baking, but this excitement was also accompanied with fear. I know my emotions at Christmas were different than what a "normal" person's would be. I was usually more thrilled about executing my plans to binge than I was about any of the other holiday festivities. The rush and power that I felt was undeniable. I felt like I was winning some type of game. The ironic thing was that the only person I was beating was myself. I now realize these emotions were all part of my self-harming addiction. I viewed the world as a place full of delicious food, and I was completely focused on how I was going to get and consume more of it.

My last week at BridgePoint was very difficult. I would soon be thrown back into the "real world", and I wasn't sure if I was ready. I definitely gained more insight on what made me tick, but I didn't know if that would be enough. Probably the most important learning was that I needed to be kinder to myself and to be more mindful of my own feelings. I didn't want to set myself up for failure, but in the same breath I knew that my behavior would eventually have to stop. That scared me, but not as much on this third visit to BridgePoint as it did before. Maybe there was hope for me this time? Until now I never realized how important *just BEING* was ... Being Aware, Being Mindful, and Being Kind to yourself. I hoped through some positive self-talk, being mindful of my surroundings, and a new awareness of my "emotional triggers" that I would be able to stop using food as a psychological crutch and eliminate my dysfunctional relationship with it. Soon it was time to say a tearful goodbye to everyone, and I was on my way home. Although somewhat nervous, I was optimistic that I had taken at least one step forward in my healing process.

HOME SWEET HOME

I arrived back home in Langenburg and was greeted by my husband and our dog Jazzie. My thoughts immediately focused on trying to figure out what Mick was thinking. Did he still have hope and love me, or had he given up? We had a long emotional chat, and he reassured me that he still cared for me and that he wasn't giving up on me yet. That was a relief, and made me instantly feel better. I was happy to be home.

I started back to work, part-time, on the Yorkton Psychiatric Unit. Was I still binging and purging? Yes, I was. Did the food control my every waking thought as before? No, it didn't. Did I get right back into my old patterns? No, I didn't. On a subconscious level, I suppose I was trying a few different things. I noticed at the end of the week that I hadn't "practiced my behavior" as much as I would have in the past. I also felt much more present than ever before. My relationship with food was much like a negative-influencing friend. A friend that was fun to be with at the time, but who always seemed to lead you into trouble eventually. Well, something was changing. I was finding that I didn't want to hang out with that friend as much. It wasn't as much fun getting into trouble with her anymore. I guess there was a light at the end of the tunnel, but I didn't see it very clearly yet.

Thinking back, I don't believe I realized that I had made some significant progress at BridgePoint because I was still occasionally purging. My thinking was so "black and white" that I didn't see any grey. However, it seemed like the *less I tried* to stop being bulimic, the *easier it got*. I'm not sure if you can understand that, as it even seems backwards when I say it aloud. *Stop trying so hard to stop … and things will get better?* That does sound really confusing, but that is how it was for me. To be present in the moment was a wonderful feeling. I really began listening to words that were spoken to me and the ones that came out of my mouth. It felt like I was in a whole new world. It was a world where what I did mattered and one where I was no longer just going through the motions of life. I remember how different I felt in those moments, like it was just yesterday, because it felt so new and so invigorating.

Was I cured of my bulimia? Not yet, I still binged, but fewer times than ever before in the past decade. Even the excitement of the binge was beginning to fade. I remember one incident in particular. I had been back from treatment for about two weeks. I was probably throwing up once per day, so still practicing the behaviour. Mick was going away for a multi-day work conference. This would have been a situation where previously, I would have been eagerly looking forward to because it meant a few days that I could binge and purge without fear of being caught. However this time, for some reason, I didn't have that familiar feeling of excitement. Almost the opposite, where I wished Mick didn't have to be away for so long. I recall wondering if something was wrong with me. How crazy does that sound? I even figured that once Mick actually left, I would find my groove. And I did. I ran to the grocery store and grabbed some munchies. Weirdly though, I didn't pick items I normally would buy. Nonetheless, it was binge food.

I got situated in front of the television and was ready to begin my feast. Again, not overly aware at the time, but I do recall now that I did not eat as much, nor as fast. The Oprah Winfrey show was on, and she was interviewing a young boy who was a drug addict. His parents said that they didn't know what to do anymore to help him. He was slowly destroying his life. The boy agreed that he needed help, and Oprah offered to send him to a rehabilitation facility. This would be his seventh admission to a treatment center, but this was his first stay at this facility. Oprah planned to follow his rehabilitation efforts.

It was time for a commercial break, so I quickly scurried to the bathroom and threw up as I didn't want to miss a minute of the show. I grabbed a big glass of water and sat back down on the couch. I found myself cheering on this young addict hoping he would get better with Oprah's help. He was only twenty-two years old and had his whole life ahead of him. This show was one of those "where are they now" episodes, and I was really interested to see how he made out. They showed clips of the young man at rehab. He had some pretty difficult days. He wanted to leave several times, but the counsellors were able to convince him to stay. Even though he had agreed to come for treatment, he was scared to lose his "vice".

It was time for another commercial break and time to purge and then get my next load of food ready. As I made my way to the bathroom something occurred to me. I hadn't eaten anything since I had thrown up during the previous commercial break. "Wow," I thought, "I must have been really wrapped up in the show." I grabbed a glass of juice after I realized that my stomach was empty.

The show resumed, and it jumped to the present day. Oprah was the only one on the stage. The audience was waiting with anticipation to see how this young man had made out. "Jeff has completed his twenty-eight day rehabilitation and is here with us today. Come on out, Jeff," Oprah said. The young man who appeared on the stage did not look like the same person who was sent to rehab. He was well-dressed, he had gained some weight, which he needed, and he had a big smile on his face. The crowd went crazy. People were clapping, cheering, and some were even crying. That is when I realized something inside me was different. I remember feeling so happy for this guy. He gave Oprah a big hug as his parents stood by with tears in their eyes. He went on to say how grateful he was that Oprah had sent him to rehab. He said that even though he had been for treatment six times before, this time was different than the others. He said that not only was the facility different this time, but more importantly he felt there was a big difference in himself. I made an instant connection to him and found myself thinking about my stays at BridgePoint. I had been there three times. The facility hadn't changed, but obviously I had. I was much more present in the moment and did not constantly focus on food. As I made these connections, I stared at the remaining food in front of me. Did I really need to finish binging on it or could I just throw it all away? That was the first time that I had ever asked myself that question.

After I threw the food away, I decided to take Jazzie for a walk. Talk about "ah-ha" moments. That was one of the biggest I have ever had. The fact that I didn't feel like I had to continue eating was a different choice for me. Replacing my coping habit with a healthier activity, such as going for a walk, was also something new. In my opinion, I was able to make different decisions because of my recent work at BridgePoint. *I was now mentally healthier to make a better choice.* I didn't have to keep being a bulimic. This may sound like a no brainer to most people, but it's not to anyone that is actively practising an addiction. So I learned … YES, there is always a choice in life, but it is not as simple and easy as it seems when you are an addict that is consumed by negative and self-harming thoughts.

The behavior of eating too much food or drinking too much alcohol is a symptom of a mental health disorder. Therefore, *the underlying mental health issue must be dealt with first, so the addict is healthier, more resilient, and is able to choose a less destructive manner to cope with their mental illness.* I also learned that my mental illness was going nowhere and neither was food, they would both still be a part of my life, so something else had to change. I had to learn to respect myself, let go of the past, and find healthier alternatives. I am certain that I would not have been able to make this change prior to the hard work I did on my mental health. Once I learned to love myself despite my flaws, it opened the door to a healthier life. Before that, I didn't respect myself enough to make better choices ... because my health didn't matter, I just wanted to numb the hurt and self-hate. I ate food to throw it up and that was just the way it was during the worst years of my addiction. I was so sick that I did not think bulimia was abnormal. In fact, is seemed very natural to me. I just lived to eat, as opposed to eating to live, for almost two decades. If that doesn't scream mental illness I'm not sure what does! How I got to that point of such an engrained illness and severe bulimia is a whole other question ... thankfully, I was eventually able to let go of wondering "why me?"

EMPTY

There's an emptiness inside
That I can't figure out
Just tell me the answer
I want to scream out

Others succeed
At things that they do
Why can't that be me?
I want to fit in too

Is it only me
Who feels this way?
It doesn't seem fair
These feelings just stay

I try different ways
To fill the void
The failed attempts
Just leave me annoyed

The need for approval
I have always had
How far do I take it?
Is this good or bad?

Many years later
The empty feeling subsides
I'm no longer the person
Who is scared and hides

A LIFE FILLED WITH COUNSELLING

June 2002 – Life continued on with many "ah-ha" moments. I was regularly visiting my counsellor and working in Yorkton. The phone rang at home one day, and our caller ID said it was the school division. I assumed the call was for Mick, but when I answered the person asked for me. I had forgotten that about a year ago I had submitted my resume to the school division, for any student counsellor positions available. There was a new opening in a neighboring community, and I was asked if I was interested in the half-time position. I was pleasantly surprised and was very interested in counselling students, so I instantly told them yes. I hung up and phoned Mick. He was excited for me. I was still a casual employee with the healthcare system in Yorkton, so I could work both jobs. I felt ready for this challenge.

After a few weeks, I felt comfortable in my new role with both the students and the school staff. More importantly, it seemed like I had a new purpose other than binging and purging. I cannot recall a single incident of binging during the workday once I became a school counsellor as it no longer consumed my thoughts. This was a big deal, as I said before, bulimia used to be my favorite friend to hang out with. Still, but less frequently, I did visit her when I was home alone, but it just wasn't as "fun" anymore. I had new priorities and was just feeling more and more present during those other activities now. It really felt like things were starting to come together for me. I felt healthier, and I wasn't getting sick as often. Thankfully, my marriage began to slowly heal as well.

ONE DAY AT A TIME

Mick and I began to try and start a family. I was hopeful every month that I wouldn't get my period, but it always arrived. I had the desire to be a mother, however I was certain that my body wasn't healthy enough to get pregnant. I had inflicted so much abuse to it over the years that I was certain that I would be cursed by the self-harm. On the positive side, I did feel healthier as I had reduced my binging and purging to about twice a month. Despite the improvements to my mental and physical health, I was very concerned about internal damage, so I decided that I should see an OB/GYN to make sure things were okay with my reproductive system.

At my appointment a few weeks later, I discussed my concerns with the doctor. He performed an internal ultrasound and told me that I had a condition called polycystic ovary syndrome. In English, that basically meant that I wasn't ovulating every month. He said that there was a good chance that I only ovulated two or three times a year.

I remember feeling like God was punishing me. Did I really deserve to be a mother when I couldn't even take care of myself for so many years? I still prayed that there was a chance to have a healthy baby. The doctor's plan was to start me on fertility medication in a couple months. This would hopefully increase my chances of conceiving.

Both Mick's parents and my own, continued to ask us when we were starting a family, so we told them about my fertility issues. I once again prayed that God would give me the strength to stay healthy. Sometimes I thought that "He" didn't want to listen to me. I didn't attend church regularly, even though I was Catholic. I expressed my faith in my own way. I tried simply to be a "good Christian". It was not so much a religion to me, but instead how I treated others ... and I always (except when focused on a binge) treated others with respect and kindness, hence the people-pleaser in me, and now I was getting better at treating myself in the same manner.

In mid-April 2003, we got a phone call from Mick's dad in Calgary. He had some bad news about my mother-in-law (who I called Mommy). She had been to the doctor several times in the last few months because of severe hip pain. She was only about sixty-four years old and seemed to always be quite healthy. She worked hard her entire life, starting with her childhood in India, and never complained about her health without good reason. Her general practitioner diagnosed her pain as a symptom of arthritis and he continued to prescribe her anti-inflammatory medication. Many months went by without any improvement. Her doctor suggested that she see a psychiatrist as he attributed her pain to depression. Our sister-in-law was also a nurse, so thankfully she decided it was time for a second opinion. Immediately, the new doctor took an X-ray of her hip. He discovered that she had a large tumor, so it required a biopsy. The tumor was the size of a grape-fruit. Basically, it had started to eat-away at her pelvis because it was cancerous. She was booked in for an urgent surgery, hopefully within the week. We dropped everything and immediately drove to Calgary. Mommy was in bed when we got to their house. She was so happy to see us that she started to cry. In her somewhat-broken English she told us, "I want to live so I can see all of my kids have children, that way, I pray to God that you get pregnant Andrea."

We stayed in Calgary for about four days, but then we had to get back to Langenburg for work. Mick's mom was sad to see us leave and was in significant pain. Her stay in the hospital would be an extensive one and she would require many hours of physio after the repairs to her hip. It would be a long road to recovery. The doctors did further tests to determine what type of cancer it was; it turned out to be multiple myeloma. Mick's younger brother and his wife lived in Calgary so they could keep us posted. Our sister-in-law had a good understanding of Mommy's medical situation since she was a nurse. She was also six months pregnant, with their first child, so that sure helped lift Mommy's spirits.

Once back in Langenburg, our local pharmacy called to tell me that my fertility medication was now in stock. With all of the medical turmoil in Calgary, I had put our fertility concerns on the back burner. It had been about two months since I saw the OB/GYN. The plan was to start the medication after my next period, which I estimated to be in a few days.

I recall this being a very hectic time for us. Mick was enrolled in a Master's Degree course and was regularly making a five hour return trip to Regina for the evening classes. Sometimes twice a week he would make the drive, immediately after work and not get home until after midnight, only to get up early the next morning to go back to work. On top of this time demand, he was always coaching some school or community sport. I was very proud of him. He managed this busy schedule along with his school administrator demands and meetings for several years ... not to mention my health issues. There were many stressors in our life during these early years of marriage, but we found a way to get through them together.

ANOTHER FALSE ALARM OR A MIRACLE?

Later that week, it was time for the annual track and field meet at Mick's high school. The weather was great, so I told Mick I would stop by and watch. I enjoyed watching the students competing in the events and visiting with parents. I decided to grab a bag of popcorn (everyone knows it is my trademark snack) and a drink. Strangely, I wasn't able to eat much of my popcorn. I had a wave of nausea that made me feel sick to my stomach. Could I be pregnant? I realized the date. My period was supposed to come today. I left the track meet and drove to the pharmacy, but instead of picking up the fertility prescription that I was supposed to begin soon, I grabbed a pregnancy test. I figured I was probably overreacting, but I wanted to make sure either way.

I went directly to the bathroom when I got home and ripped open the box. I put the stick on the bathroom counter and walked away, already counting the seconds in my head. I waited an extra couple of minutes just to make sure. I looked at the stick on the counter and saw two bright pink lines. I thought there must be something wrong. I couldn't be pregnant. I hadn't even started my fertility meds yet. It was 3:15 p.m., so I still had time to see the doctor for a second opinion. Luckily, I was able to drop in. Mick had a class in Regina that night, so I knew he would be leaving right away. I called him at work and told him to meet me at the doctor's office. I'm not sure if I believed in miracles before this day, but I became a believer that day … the doctor confirmed it, I was pregnant!

Most women are ecstatic when they find out they are having a baby, especially if they had been trying for a while. There were so many emotions running through my mind. Was I happy? Of course. Was I scared? Absolutely … I was scared out of my mind. It all happened so quickly, that I started to cry in the office. Tears of joy, tears of relief, tears of fear. My doctor asked me how I felt. I honestly didn't know if I could handle nine months of taking care of myself. So many thoughts rushed through my head. I knew I would have to stop drinking, stop smoking, and completely block out thoughts of binging and purging. My doctor reassured me that I would be just fine. I had my doubts.

After about twenty minutes of sharing our joint excitement, and my fears, Mick had to leave for his class in Regina. Just before he left, we called his mom in Calgary to tell her that her prayers had been answered. "That way I pray and God heard me," she said. She was very excited for us. I called my parents next to tell them the shocking news, and they were as equally excited for us. There hadn't been a baby on my side of the family for many years.

Over the next few days, I felt overwhelmed with just about everything. I felt the pressure was on to be a "good" pregnant lady. Cutting out the alcohol wouldn't be hard, but cigarette smoking would definitely be tough. And then there was the food. Even though I reduced my incidents of purging significantly, how in the world was I going to be able to quit my bulimia habits cold turkey? Nutrition was essential for my unborn baby. I talked to my friend Debbie. She had faith in me. She said that I would instinctively know what to do. Women get pregnant all the time, so why should my pregnancy be any different? Well, for starters, most "normal" women aren't "recovering" from a severe eating disorder or continually battling with severe body image concerns. Currently I was at a comfortable weight, but how would I feel when I started gaining maternity weight? Would I feel the urge to binge and purge? If I did, then how would that effect the baby? I needed to wrap my head around all the "what if" questions that were going through my head. My mom was always there when I needed to chat and Mick understood me better than anyone, so I knew I could count on both of them. I told myself that I would have no secrets and talk to my supports when I was feeling overwhelmed. My pregnancy was definitely a pivotal "turning point". Now I had more to care for other than myself. It stressed me out, but I learned to take one day at a time and keep my lines of communication open with my counsellor, my friend Debbie, my mom, and Mick.

ALONE IN A CROWD

In a crowd
I'm all alone
A smile I show
To set the tone

Words are spoken
Which I don't hear
I nod to agree
To avoid the fear

I worry about things
I like to hide
To tell the truth
Would disturb the tide

This was my way
For many years
And the feelings inside
Have brought many tears

But now I am present
When I'm in a crowd
To talk and laugh
I am finally allowed

My journey continues
With each waking day
One step at a time
Has become my new way

SUMMER HOLIDAYS ... VEGAS "BABY"!

A few months later, Mick and I were off to Vegas with a couple of our best friends, Kelly and Christine. We were really looking forward to the trip because Christine and I had tickets to a Céline Dion concert. We drove about two thousand kilometres, so you can imagine all the pee breaks ... with a couple girls in the car and one of them being pregnant. I didn't really feel that pregnant yet. I guess I didn't know what to expect. Even though Mick didn't like it, I was still casually smoking, but much less than before. I was trying to cut myself a little slack. My main goal was not to get too ahead of myself and just take things one day at a time. I was peeing more than usual, so I assumed that was a good sign. My boobs seemed to be getting bigger and were sore. Yet, once we arrived, the fun began. Vegas was crazy hot, as it was the middle of July, so we spent most of the day in the pool and in the air conditioned casinos and malls. The thermometer read around forty-five degrees Celsius on most days ... well above one hundred ten degrees Fahrenheit!

I clearly remember our first meal. I was experiencing a fair amount of nausea, but not to the point of vomiting. If you've ever been to Vegas then you know all about their amazing buffets. You would think that an "All You Can Eat" joint wasn't the greatest choice for someone trying to overcome an eating disorder. However, you can't avoid food in your life like you can alcohol or cigarettes. Thankfully, I wasn't having the same urges to overeat as in the past. I only ate moderate amounts during the trip, but something was definitely different with my outlook towards food. I found myself taking my time to chew and really taste the food. I had this whole new sense of smell and taste. I also stayed clear of the sweets and really rich foods. This was new for me. Not that I was deliberately depriving myself, but I just didn't feel like eating those foods anymore. It was another "ah-ha" moment. I remember being in the moment and being able to take in all the wonderful sights, tastes, and smells around us. The weather was beautiful and the pool was refreshing. We were having so much fun with our dear friends. Christine and I became really good friends over the last couple years, while Kelly and Mick had been buddies since he moved to Langenburg. Now, as couples, we enjoyed many laughs and evenings out together. That being said, I can't recall if I had told Christine about my eating disorder at this point yet. I want to say yes, but I'm not totally sure. Either way, I always knew Christine had my back.

Céline Dion put on a spectacular show, and we both had some teary moments during the show. The whole trip was memorable. To this day we occasionally laugh our asses off when reliving the Vegas trip. Our treacherous ride through the mountains in our little car (the Vibe), almost hitting a buffalo, and checking into a grungy Bear Camp Motel in the middle of "Nowhere" Yellowstone National Park (just because Mick wanted to take a five hour detour to see Old Faithful) are all wonderful memories. It goes to show you that life truly is more about the people you are with, and the journey you take together, rather than the destination of the trip.

The rest of the summer flew by, including our time in Calgary. Mick's younger brother and his wife welcomed a baby boy into their family and my mother-in-law was in less pain. She had finished her chemo sessions and was recovering quite well from her hip surgery. I wasn't showing much yet, as I was only about three months along. Surprisingly, I think I was beginning to look forward to having a baby bump, especially after seeing our new nephew arrive.

BABY-BUMP BODY IMAGE

The school year began, and I was happy to be back at work. I worked a few days at the hospital over the summer, but we were away from home for most of it. Some of my co-workers at the school commented how I was beginning to show, and they were right. There was a new doctor in town, so we booked an appointment and heard the baby's heartbeat for the first time. It was an incredible experience. There was a life growing inside of me that we had created. Our first ultrasound in Yorkton was a little scary, as I recall my concern and hope that everything was okay with the baby. I also set up an appointment with an OB/GYN in Regina as we decided we would deliver there in case there were any complications. Also, that would allow me to stay with my parents as we approached the due date of January 28, 2004.

I'm not sure how many pivotal "turning points" I'm allowed to have in my road to recovery, but the next one was about a month later when I felt my baby kick for the first time. That was one of the most unique feelings I have ever felt. I can't explain the emotion it created. It was like a switch flipped on in my brain, and I truly realized that I was going to be a mom, ready or not. I realized that I needed to take care of myself in order to take care of our baby. Food became food that I ate to live, and slowly but surely that became its purpose for me. My confidence grew and I now felt that I was healthy enough to manage this new responsibility. That sure was a good feeling.

I was around sixteen weeks along when I had my next ultrasound appointment in Regina. Mick and I decided to find out the sex of the baby. The technician said they usually don't like to share the sex at that point because they usually cannot be one hundred percent certain. Minutes after examining the evidence, the technician told us that she was quite sure that we were going to have a boy. She laughed and joked, "It seems like your little fellow is posing for Mom and Dad!"

I began wearing maternity clothes around the four and a half month mark. I was enjoying the initial weight gain, which of course is ironic. I had spent about sixteen years being obsessed with food, numbers on scales, every pound I gained, and yet here I was celebrating my weight gain each week. Wherever a pregnant woman goes her weight seems to be a topic of discussion, whether it's at the doctor's office or just chatting with family, friends, and colleagues. Someone always seems to be commenting on your weight. It is about the only time that people can talk about "how big you are getting" without feeling guilty about their comments. People definitely let you know when you are getting "huge"! I charted everything from my weight gain, to my food likes and dislikes, to how I felt emotionally. I wasn't eating that much more than usual (meaning in my post-bulimic diet), yet I gained about thirty pounds by my fifth month. The baby was kicking up a storm, and I loved it.

Fast forward to around mid-December, and I was enormous! I was gaining weight all over my body, not just in my belly. My local physician concluded that I would not carry to term. My blood pressure was up a bit, but it was still okay. My doctor predicted that our boy would come on January 9, 2004, which was three weeks before my due date. He wished me well in Regina as he would not see me until after I had the baby and once we returned home. Mick and I headed into Regina for Christmas, and the plan was that I would stay there until I delivered the baby.

A DIFFERENT KIND OF CHRISTMAS
AND AN AMAZING PRESENT

This Christmas was quite different than any holiday season that I could remember for quite some time. First of all, I was pregnant. Secondly, I weighed the most I ever had in my life, but more importantly, I didn't feel the stress of food. I wasn't planning how many times I would binge and purge either. I may not have fully recognized the extent of the change in my thinking at that time, but I sure can see it now.

My brother's wife was expecting too. She was due in April, so there were many things to be thankful for this Christmas. My parents would have two new grandchildren soon. I was feeling humungous by this point. My legs were swelling, and the heartburn was endless. Even though my belly was huge, I did notice that I could push in on it. There seemed to be a bit more room in there than what the baby was taking up. Nothing alarming, but throughout much of my pregnancy, I also had many episodes of Braxton-Hicks contractions. Over the holidays Mick went to Calgary for a few days to see his family. His mom was in remission, but the past year had been a rough one for her. Cancer, in the form of multiple myeloma, attacked many of her bone sites. It also depleted her immune system. Yet, she was a very tough lady and my father-in-law was by her side since her diagnosis.

By New Year's Eve, Mick was back in Regina. We celebrated my birthday on the third of January and then he returned to Langenburg. Our plan was that he would work until I notified him that I was in labor. That phone call was made on January 8. Earlier that evening I was out on a drive with my parents. We were looking at the Christmas light displays in the city park when the cramps began. My mom said to keep track of them so we could tell if I getting them regularly. The cramps occurred about every thirty minutes. I suspected it was false labor. Once we got back I tried to relax by watching some television, but the "cramps" kept coming. I phoned the hospital and the nurse suggested that I have a warm bath, monitor my cramps, and call back if they continued for an extended period of time. I laid in the tub and watched my baby bump twist and turn. This baby sure liked the warm water. I dried myself off and felt a little better as the intensity of the cramps seemed to lessen.

By 10:00 p.m. the cramps came back with vengeance. I called Mick. I wasn't due for another three weeks, so he thought it was most likely a false alarm. I tried to convince myself he was right. However, I wasn't totally convinced as I laid in bed groaning beside my mother for the next six hours. Mom tracked the time of every "cramp" until she fell asleep on me. I got out of bed and rocked back and forth in my parents' rocking chair. I began to worry that I really was in labor as the cramps hit every fifteen minutes. I called the hospital and they told me to come in for an assessment. I woke up my mom and told her we better go to the hospital. It was about 4:00 a.m. when my parents helped me into the car and called Mick. They told him they would update him once we knew more. I was admitted into the hospital and was given something for the pain. The doctor told me I was only dilated a single centimeter. I couldn't believe it. "Holy shit," I thought. "I have nine more centimeters to go?" I tried to rest, but couldn't. The contractions hurt too much. A nurse took my vital signs and found that my blood pressure was elevated. At about 8:00 a.m. the doctor assessed me again. She was not happy with my elevated BP. She gave me some medication to encourage the contractions and said to give Mick a call to tell him that the baby would be delivered today. Mick got that call at about 8:30 a.m. and was at the hospital in Regina by 11:00 a.m.

The next six hours were kind of a blur, but I do remember my water breaking and then things progressed quite quickly. Our son, Ajay, was born at 4:30 p.m. weighing just over five pounds on January 9, just like my local GP had predicted. The nurse said that it looked like Ajay had been in the oven a bit too long, because his skin seemed a bit loose on his arms and legs, kind of like you would see on an old man who has lost his muscle tone. The "overdone" look was a bit odd because he was premature by three weeks. All along I was given the impression that he would be a large baby. Nevertheless, I held him for a couple minutes and cried with joy. Mick showed him off to my parents, Auntie Kim, and Uncle Geoff. He was beautiful.

THE HAZE OF AFTERBIRTH

After delivering Ajay, things got really fuzzy. I needed to get about forty stitches because I had torn quite badly. My stomach hurt, and I was so very tired. Once the doctor finished with me I wanted to go see my new baby. I was helped into the wheelchair, and Mick took me to the neonatal unit. I saw my little boy in the incubator with wires all over him. I stood up out of the wheelchair and everything went black. The next thing I remember was waking up in labor and delivery feeling like crap. I had fainted. My hemoglobin was quite low because I had lost a significant amount of blood delivering the baby. I needed to rest, and Mick reassured me that our baby boy was fine.

The next day Mick told me that the nurses in the neonatal unit commented about Ajay's little fists being clenched. They asked him if I was taking Paxil, an anti-depressant. Mick replied, "Yes." I had been prescribed it throughout my pregnancy and my doctors assured me that it was safe. The nurse explained to Mick that they see numerous "Paxil babies" in neonatal. She said it was fairly common to see some "tremors and fist-clenching" in these babies. I guess I wasn't the only pregnant woman taking an antidepressant. The tremors were a sign of the drug leaving the baby's system. I guess it makes sense. If a mother is taking a prescription or an illegal drug during pregnancy, the baby has no choice but to ingest some as well. This concerned Mick, but the doctor reassured him that in a few days Ajay would stop trembling, and he would be just fine.

The next day I got moved to the maternity unit. I was put on an iron supplement, and they monitored my BP. When I spoke to the doctor, I was told that my baby and I had suffered from placental abruption. That meant my placenta started to rip away from the uterine lining. I had none of the classic symptoms pre-delivery so it went undetected. I had no external bleeding before Ajay was born, so the blood simply collected in my uterus – another reason why I had lost so much blood during delivery. The doctor said it was about fifty percent torn, so Ajay hadn't been getting sufficient nutrients since the abruption, but thankfully enough oxygen. The doctor estimated that the baby had lost three to four pounds inside of me. "It's good that you went into labor when you did," the doctor said. I knew exactly what he was saying. It was fortunate that my baby came out kicking earlier than his due date, otherwise oxygen depletion would have resulted. Thank God our little Ajay was a fighter.

Ajay stayed in neonatal for six days, and I was back to my parents' house after the fourth day. I still felt very sore, but had a post-birth adrenaline surge. I couldn't stop thinking about Ajay. He really was a miracle. Sadly, there was a girl that Mick knew who delivered a still-born just weeks prior. Mick didn't tell me about her loss while I was pregnant, as he did not want me to be concerned. The cause of her loss, unfortunately, was placental abruption.

I spent most of the day with Ajay while he was in the hospital. I felt a bit like a failure because breastfeeding wasn't working for me. I began pumping and bottle feeding. Once again, Mick had to get back to work, but would come back on Friday. After six days in neonatal, we brought Ajay to my mom and dad's house. I stayed there for a week just to get a little help before heading home to Langenburg. It was both exciting and scary … I was finally a mother.

My discharge plan included several visits by the public health nurse. During her initial visit I mentioned to the nurse that I was still bleeding quite a bit and that things just didn't feel right. Oddly, she never performed a physical examination during any of these appointments. Instead, she simply reassured me that the pain was probably due to my post-delivery stitches. Nevertheless, her reassurance didn't comfort me too much. Physically, I felt terrible. I had also mentioned to the nurse that my hemoglobin levels were quite low, about seventy-six, upon discharge from the hospital. Therefore, the constant blood loss concerned me. I undoubtedly was functioning on adrenaline. Approximately eight days post-delivery, and about two hours after another homecare visit by the nurse, I told Mom that I was going to run to the store. Instead, I drove myself to the nearest walk-in clinic as I was very concerned by the feeling that something was falling out of my crotch. I know some readers may not want to hear any of the after-birth details, but why stop now? I have already shared the gory details of my purging episodes, so I presume a few childbirth details can't be that much worse!

When I got to the clinic, I quickly told them why I was there. The clinic's nurse checked on me and commented on the yellow color of my skin. I replied, "I had a baby eight days ago, and lost a lot of blood. I'm still bleeding and some of the clots are pretty big." The doctor came in, and I gave him the run down too. I was laying on the table, and he asked me to spread my legs. Honest to God, he didn't even touch me. He just closed my legs back up and told me to go straight to the Emergency Unit. He said he was phoning the OB/GYN on call to meet me there. "Who drove you here?" he asked. "I drove myself," I said. He couldn't believe it. I told him I would go straight to my parents' and someone would drive me to the Emergency Unit from there.

I left the clinic and started to shake. I actually had to hold my crotch because it felt like I was going to burst. I got back to my parents', and I was a blubbering fool. "Mom, you have to take me to the hospital right now. I just came back from the clinic, and I need to get to the hospital to see the OB/GYN." My mom and dad didn't know what the heck was going on. I filled them in, and my mom got me in the car. I had pre-pumped baby bottles in the fridge for Ajay. My dad and sister stayed home to take care of him.

The Emergency nurse knew exactly who I was when we walked in. The specialist was waiting for me too. I went to the examination room and next thing I knew I had a shot of Demerol in my leg. I'll be careful and try not to be too graphic. Basically, the doctor removed the blood clots and the rest of the placenta that was still in my body since giving birth eight days ago. It wasn't the most pleasant medical procedure I've ever had done that is for sure. Afterwards, he sent me home, but I was scheduled for an ultrasound first thing the next morning. After they looked at my ultrasound, I ended up having an emergency D&C as there were still more fragments of the placenta that needed to be removed. What a crazy and painful couple of days that was, but I would do it all over again as long as my baby was healthy … and he was.

MOTHERHOOD – AM I STRONG ENOUGH?

Some of you may be wondering why my storyline has shifted away from disordered eating and what do all these details regarding pregnancy and childbirth have to do with my eating disorder. Here is the honest truth. I never thought I would be able to have children for two main reasons. First, I was pretty certain that I had done so much damage to my body that I could not even get pregnant, let alone deliver a healthy baby. This left me wondering … Was I healthy enough to bear children? Would my electrolyte levels ever get back to normal ranges? How much damage had I done to my abdomen? I had thrown up thousands of times as a young adult, so I was sure that my addiction would haunt me later in life.

Secondly, I told myself over and over again that I would not make a good mother. I couldn't even take care of myself for many years, so how could I expect that I was capable of taking care of a baby? What about the weight gain during pregnancy, would I obsess over that? I was very aware of my triggers and gaining weight was a big one. I definitely did not want to revert to my bulimic mentality or behaviors because I couldn't handle the weight gain.

In total, I gained eighty pounds during my pregnancy with Ajay. I was 112 pounds when I got pregnant and 192 pounds on the day I delivered. It didn't bother me so much when I was pregnant, but I wondered if I would be okay with my larger size after delivering the baby … I knew baby weight does not disappear overnight, unless you are a celebrity or a fitness fanatic that sheds weight quickly … which I definitely was not.

Ajay kept us pretty busy with feedings, every two to three hours for the first four months. I still couldn't believe he was my baby. To my surprise, my motherly instincts kicked in and so did my confidence. We flew to Calgary when Ajay was three months old so he could meet Mick's family. My in-laws had a big traditional party to welcome Ajay to the family. My mother-in-law was so happy. She was still in remission, so she was feeling much better and had the energy to hold and play with Ajay. That was incredible to watch.

The next few months were filled with plenty of "firsts" from Ajay. These moments seemed to keep me distracted from my weight. However, I did have a few cries wondering if I would ever get back to my average weight of 115-pounds. As a result, motherhood was filled with many emotional ups and downs. Despite the anxiety caused by my body-image concerns, *I never did binge and purge again.*

THIS IS JUST CRAZY

Summer was here before we knew it, and Mick continued taking university classes, so we spent a big chunk of July in Regina. My parents loved having us there as they got to spoil Ajay. A couple weeks into the summer, I started feeling a bit sick, but didn't think too much of it. One evening, while we were out for supper with my brother Geoff and sister-in-law Shannon, I mentioned that I felt a bit nauseated. Shannon joked, "Maybe you're pregnant again!" I laughed it off with, "Yeah, right!" I wasn't quite ready for all that again considering the recent delivery complications. I was due to get my period soon, so I figured that was why I felt so sick to my stomach.

Three days later I found myself at the store buying a pregnancy test just to rule out Shannon's hunch. Shockingly, the test was positive! Many of the same emotions rushed through my mind ... times ten! I hadn't even lost all the baby weight that I had gained with Ajay, and here I was pregnant again. I now weighed about 125 pounds and my regular clothes almost fit me again. This was just crazy! I wondered how in the world I would ever manage two infants born about a year apart while Mick was working, coaching on the weekends, and completing his degree in the evenings. Talk about anxiety!

To make sure the test was accurate, I ran over to the walk-in medical clinic. Ironically, it was the same clinic that I ran to after Ajay was born. I gave a urine sample, and the doctor came into the room and told me I was indeed pregnant. "But I can't be. I have a six-month-old baby at home." The doctor looked at me puzzled. "Did you and your husband have sex recently?" he asked. Obviously we had, but only a few times in the last couple months. I also told him about my polycystic ovary syndrome, which was supposed to make it really difficult to get pregnant. "Well I guess it's a miracle then!" he said with a chuckle.

I stopped at a store on the way home and got Mick a greeting card, with a picture of a baby's foot on the cover and a personal note on the inside, to deliver him the surprising news. After he read the card he was speechless. Once the shock wore off, he was ecstatic. This truly was a miracle. I didn't think I could get pregnant even once, let alone a second time without even trying. It was time for me to step up to the plate once again and make sure our new baby was healthy just like our first.

By three months, I started to prominently show again. I guess I had a head start with a "Mommy tummy" already in place. I was considered high risk because of the placental abruption issue we had with Ajay. We planned to have the baby in Regina with the doctor who helped deliver Ajay. My family doctor monitored me closely as well. My due date was April 6, 2005. Friends couldn't believe how big I already was. By the time I was five months pregnant, I looked like I was eight months. Really not a great image for a "non-active" bulimic to see when she looks in the mirror. My legs were also starting to swell. I guess they just matched the rest of me. I was still taking my anti-depressant, Paxil, which was still considered safe by doctors at the time. My blood pressure was also being monitored because of the pre-delivery concerns with Ajay. I was managing being a mom and being pregnant, but I was exhausted. Mick was so busy with all of his demands as well, but always helped out when he could.

It was February, and my April due date started to creep up on us. A friend from Langenburg was going into Regina, so I decided that Ajay, Jazzie, and I would catch a lift in with her as I had appointments with my OB/GYN. We arrived in Regina and settled in at my folks' place. I was glad to see my doctor, because I was noticing a significant change in my medical situation over the past week. Kim took me to my appointment, and the first thing the nurse had me do was step on the weight scale. I removed my dad's slippers that I was wearing because my feet were so swollen. I was afraid to look at the scale because I was enormous! My legs and feet were so fat that they felt like they were going to explode. Once the nurse completed a few measurements I was sent into the doctor's office.

"How do you feel Andrea?" the doctor asked and then continued, "I can't imagine very good because you have gained twenty pounds in the past week." She rechecked my blood pressure, and it was high. I think it was around 145/95. I told her I was quite uncomfortable lately and that my heartburn was awful during the night. "I really can't imagine feeling like this for another month and a half," I told her. The doctor recommended that I be admitted to the hospital so they could monitor my blood pressure and complete another ultrasound.

I have to admit, honestly, I was pretty scared. Ajay had been our little miracle baby, so I feared that there was something definitely wrong with me or the baby this time. Why had I gained so much weight recently and so quickly? It definitely wasn't because of over-eating. I hadn't eaten very much because it physically felt like I didn't have any room in my stomach. My abdomen area felt very crowded and I slept sitting up most nights because of the heartburn. My whole body felt like a big fat sausage swelling on the barbecue. Once again, not a great feeling for someone with a history of an eating disorder.

Kim helped me "get a grip" on the situation and my anxiousness. She informed my parents while I grabbed my things and gave Mick a quick call. I hoped my vital signs would return to normal with a little rest in the hospital. Once admitted, I was sent for the ultrasound. Much like my last pregnancy, they questioned me about my due date. "Your baby is measuring quite large for your due date. His head is larger than the normal range based on the due date." This terrified me. I wondered why his head was so big. "That could mean encephalitis," I thought. I verbalized my concern to the tech, "When you say that his head seems too large what exactly does that mean? I am pretty sure on my dates, so is there something wrong?" I knew that he wasn't allowed to say too much, but since he was asking me those questions I figured he could at least reassure me that everything was okay. The technician replied, "There is no reason to worry, he is just going to be a big baby. The size of your baby's head, in relation to the rest of his body, is not alarming. Your doctor will discuss the ultrasound with you once she has reviewed it." I felt a bit better after hearing that, but I still wondered why my blood pressure was so high.

I woke up the next morning, and the nurse checked my vitals. To my relief, my blood pressure had come down and the bloodwork results looked fine. My doctor sent me home to rest, but wanted me to keep my BP down. That may have been impossible with a one-year-old waiting for me at home. Granted, I was very thankful that I had the help of my family right now, but I wasn't going to just sit around and do nothing for the next six weeks. I knew the doctor was right though, as it was getting quite difficult for me to breathe deeply and to walk around.

Saturday, March 5, 2005. I came down the stairs that morning, and by the time I got to the kitchen I was out of breath. My parents were just out the door to spend a few nights at the Moose Jaw Spa, a trip they had planned several months ago. My mom noticed my breathing difficulties and how shiny the skin looked on my legs. She encouraged me to let Kim take care of Ajay and told me to rest. "Maybe you should get Kim to check your blood pressure with my machine," she hollered as they left. Later that day, I sat down at the table and Kim got out the BP machine. She put the cuff around my arm and pushed the button. We anxiously waited for the reading to appear. Ajay sat watching with us as the machine went "beep, beep" and the reading appeared ... 160/110 ... that was not a good number. Kim told me to get ready because she was taking me to the Emergency unit. She informed my parents by phone, but told them not to worry. I didn't see the situation as alarming, but figured it was the best plan just in case.

When we got to the ER they sent me right in after I told them what was going on. "Oh I'm sure the reading on my mom's machine was wrong. I bet my BP is probably normal." I seemed to have a habit of either overreacting or making light of things, instead of taking things in stride for what they were ... good or bad. My mom often told me that people may not take me seriously if I always make jokes during tense situations just to lighten the mood. So anyways, while I was busy blubbering to the nurse that everything was probably fine, she had already measured my blood pressure. She removed the cuff and called for the doctor. It was 175/110 and my pulse rate was 110. That shut me up rather quickly.

I was admitted into the hospital within the hour. Kim took Ajay back home and said she would call Mick in Langenburg to let him know what had transpired. I was taken for another ultrasound, which included the, "Are you sure on your dates?" question again. Another blood test and urine sample too. After I was returned to my room the doctor came in to check on me. The plan was that I would spend the rest of the day and night in the hospital. They gave me an antihypertensive pill and would check my vitals in the morning. Kim came back after dropping Ajay off at my brother's house. I was starting to get a little concerned by this point, I guess my joking around wasn't a solution to bringing down my blood pressure after all.

It was also kind of a coincidence that it was March 5. I had told Mick months ago that this baby would be early much like Ajay. I guessed that I would deliver about a month early, so March 6 and not April 6 as expected. Mick reminded me of this when we spoke later that evening. He kidded that I was probably just trying to win our bet by having the baby this week.

READY OR NOT ... IT'S HAPPENING!

I remember falling asleep around 9:00 p.m. that evening and not waking up until seven the next morning. I rarely slept straight through the night, so I must have been really tired. Another thing that seemed weird was that I didn't get up to go to the bathroom all night either. Actually, I didn't feel the urge to go pee even after waking up. I sat up in the bed and had a sip of water. I had a brutal headache, almost like a bad hangover. About five minutes later, the doctor came in with his entourage. He asked me how I slept and I told him that I had a great sleep. I jokingly said, "I didn't even get up to pee last night, so maybe that's why I slept so well." The cuff on my arm was inflated and it got quite tight around my arm before it finally started deflating. Of course, I wasn't in any state to make sense of the obvious as I glanced over at the numbers on the machine. I don't remember the exact readings, but they were very high. "Okay, so that can't be good," I joked again. The doctor was asking me a few questions when I began to see a bunch of sparkles floating all over the room. I told him what I saw and that I had a headache. "Well, we got the test results back and your urine is full of protein. Your bloodwork concerns me as well," the doctor said. "Basically, we think your kidneys are starting to shut down so we are sending you to labor and delivery to be induced. You will be having your baby today as that is the only way to treat your condition."

What? This was all happening so fast. What about my husband? Would Mick get here in time? When the doctor said that they were sending me to be induced he meant right then and there. Kim had fortunately arrived while I was being seen by the doctor. She asked the doctor if she could accompany me while I was being induced, and I asked the nurse if she could call my husband in Langenburg. The nurse said we could call him right now. Mick picked up the phone after the second ring. I must have sounded like a complete basket case, but I guess that was to be expected. Mick was playing in a hockey tournament that weekend, and he was just getting ready to go to his game. Instead of me trying to explain to him what was happening, I just handed the phone to the nurse.

"Hi Mick, this is Andrea's nurse. Yes, that's correct. She is going to be induced right away. No, I don't think you should play your hockey game. Yes, I think you have time for a quick shower before you leave," said the nurse. She started laughing as she hung up the phone. "Your husband is hilarious. He was wondering if he could sneak a hockey game in before you go into labor." Ask me if I was surprised. Kim and I both laughed. "Yeah, that's my brother-in-law for you," Kim said.

Our laughter came to a halt about thirty minutes later. The nurse warned me that I would feel the contractions come on pretty fast after the induction. She was right. She explained that when a mother is induced prematurely, the pain can be intense. Basically, what would naturally happen over a course of weeks was happening in a day. The baby was not in the proper position for delivery, but we were making him come out, ready or not!

Mick obviously figured out the urgency of the situation and hustled his butt to Regina. He arrived about 1:00 p.m., and I was relieved to see him. Kim brought Ajay up to the hospital, and my parents were returning from Moose Jaw. The contractions were so painful, even more so than with Ajay. It was about six hours since I had been induced, and I was trying to distract myself with the ongoing conversation that Kim and Mick were having. Ajay was too young to understand why Mommy was moaning like an animal caught in a hunter's trap. A bit later, Mick and I walked to my new room in labor and delivery. Judging by the way I felt, I was certain that I was ready to start pushing. "You have dilated to one centimeter," the doctor said. I clearly wasn't ready to deliver yet. About twenty minutes later I got up to go to the bathroom. I remember having a familiar sensation and then my water broke, partially on my husband's shoes! Mick wiped off his shoes while chuckling at my aim and then called for the nurse. I got back into bed and the nurse checked on me. Surprisingly, I was now dilated to four centimeters.

The next few hours were the worst. I felt like giving up at one point, well maybe a few times. I'm sure many moms out there can relate to what I mean. What I do remember, or maybe I should say what I don't remember was hearing my baby cry when he finally came out. For some reason, unlike Ajay, this baby did not respond with any sort of noise whatsoever. Instead, I heard over the intercom, "Respiratory stat in labor and delivery," loudly repeated three times. A few more doctors and nurses hustled into the room. As I write these words, I can feel my heart beating faster as I recall this memory. As I laid there, I instantly forgot about my pain and just wanted to know if my baby was okay. Mick came to my side and reassured me. The doctor informed us that the baby wasn't breathing for a brief moment, but reassured us that everything should be fine now. I hoped and prayed that I could believe him. I didn't get a full sense of relief until I got to hold the newest addition to the family ... Sammy ... our beautiful baby boy!

We couldn't snuggle him long as the medical staff needed to take him to the NICU to have some tests done even though he was a healthy weight of seven pounds six ounces. Unfortunately, Sammy had a seizure shortly after he was born so they wanted to ensure that it was not due to anything too serious. I remember seeing Sammy in the incubator with the wires hooked up and intravenous lines in the scalp of his head. The director of the NICU had spoken to us earlier, so we knew that he would be admitted into the unit simply because he was premature. However, we were now concerned about why he had a seizure. Sammy, once again much like Ajay, was a "Paxil baby" according to the nurses. His fists were somewhat clenched as well, but the tremors were not quite as evident as they were with his older brother.

There were so many little preemies on the unit. If you removed the intravenous lines, the nasal gastric tube, and all the wires from him, Sammy didn't look like he belonged in the unit. The average weight of the babies in NICU was only about three pounds. At over seven pounds, Sammy definitely raised the average weight in the unit. The doctor explained the tests that Sammy would undergo. His lungs were healthy for being a premature baby, but they needed to rule out some concerns related to the seizure. He was being fed through a nasal gastric tube for now, plus he was jaundiced. It sounded like he would be in the unit longer than Ajay, even though he was a larger baby. As far as my health, I actually felt much better than I did after Ajay was born. The labor and delivery had been very painful, but it ended there. My blood work was all good, so that was encouraging news.

Sammy stayed in the neonatal unit for almost ten days. All of his tests came back normal. We were so happy to have a second healthy boy. The intravenous site had been changed about four times, so his head was shaved in several spots. We asked the nurse to trim his hair on the other side too in order to even it out, so Sammy ended up coming home with a cute little Mohawk haircut. This time around my weight started coming off more rapidly. I think I had already lost about forty pounds by the time Sammy was released from the hospital. I could actually see my ankles again!

I recall being very grateful, as I had two healthy babies despite the abuse I had inflicted on my body for so many years. I'm not sure if I was just lucky, or if someone was looking out for us, or if I had changed my self-harming behaviors just in time. I was so thankful that I was able to safely deliver our two wonderful gifts into this world. No matter what the reason was for our good fortune, I promised myself that I was never going back to my old ways now that I had this greater responsibility and purpose of being a mother.

LOVE YOURSELF

When we met I thought he wouldn't like me
As my baggage would no doubt come with a fee
I was a girl that was just looking for true love
So was this the person YOU sent me from above?

Then the day came, he asked me to be his wife
Yes I said, and we eagerly began our new life
The honeymoon ended, and then my fears set in
The real me had surfaced, it felt like such a sin

The deception began, and many lies I did tell
I prayed he would love me, despite my hell

Life got messy, and occasionally quite cruel
It wasn't long before I looked like the fool

But then the healing began, with him by my side
Thank God he stuck around, for this bumpy ride
Years have gone by, we're blessed with two boys
Days of deception, are now filled with life's joys

I know that he loves me that is easy to see
The question I need to ask is do I love me?
My answer is finally Yes, I do love myself
Which helps put past demons, on the shelf

A NEW CHAPTER BEGINS

Our new family returned to Langenburg shortly after Sammy was discharged. Mick's parents could hardly wait for us to come to Calgary. I believe Mommy was still in remission at this time. I say I think, because it's hard for me to remember exact timelines when it came to her fight with cancer. She was either in the hospital or rehabilitation center more than she was at home during her ongoing medical battle. Either way, we definitely planned to visit Calgary in early July.

I soon began to settle into my new routine with two children born within thirteen months of each other. Sammy was a good baby, which definitely helped. Ajay didn't start walking until he was almost eighteen months, so I often had two babies to carry around. I guess that helped me get back in shape. The spring was beautiful that year, so I went for daily walks with the boys in their double stroller. I loved my new family.

Mick completed his Master's Degree later that spring. I was relieved because it would lighten his extremely busy schedule so that he could have more free time to be with his family. In addition, I knew Mick was thrilled that both of his boys could attend his graduation ceremony ... that made it all worth it. Almost everything Mick did was for his boys and me. I was so proud of all the hard work he had put in. Mick returned the compliment to me by saying how proud he was of me for holding the household, and my recovery, together over the extremely busy past year. His words of appreciation meant the world to me and they encouraged me to keep up the fight. I now knew that I would be okay.

Calgary Grammy and Papa were thrilled with their new grandson when they met him that summer. Everything seemed to be going well in my life. My children were healthy, I was healthy, and my husband completed his degree. Things were definitely on an upward swing. Even most of the weight I had gained during my pregnancy came off. My blood pressure was still moderately high, so I continued monitoring it. Otherwise, I felt pretty good physically and mentally. To think that I had spent over fifteen years with my head in a toilet seemed like a bizarre dream. I was amazed at how far I had come in the past two years. Food had become food again. I ate very healthy by choice. Sweets weren't very appealing to me, so it wasn't hard to avoid them. People commented on how good I looked after having two children born so recently ... I appreciated that, but I didn't obsess over it as I had in the past. When I think about it, I had gained and lost about one hundred fifty pounds in less than two years. The most amazing part was that I didn't revert to my old ways. Even though I had two difficult pregnancies, I survived and came out the other end mentally stronger and physically healthier than ever before.

Every once in a while, but not very often, when Mick complains that he is "so sick", I remind him about the size of Sammy's head and where it came out of ... I honestly think, that if men had to have the babies, like give actual birth, there wouldn't be very many children in the world. I think the woman's role in child bearing should be applauded and recognized because of the hardships our bodies go through during the pregnancy and birth of these beautiful little miracles we have created.

CAN I KEEP IT ALL TOGETHER?

The next several years had many different hurdles, both small and big, but in most cases I amazed myself by how well I handled them in comparison to the past. My new confidence to overcome the new challenges that would have "emotionally crushed" me in years prior was a great new feeling. "Life can't be this easy, can it?" I asked myself. It wasn't long until some larger hurdles appeared to put my new resolve to the test.

I returned to work on the Pine Unit in Yorkton when Sammy was about five months old, as I didn't qualify for maternity leave benefits due to the close proximity of my delivery dates. I regularly had my blood pressure checked, it was still moderately elevated on a consistent basis. My periods returned to normal, but for some reason I was experiencing significant pain in the first few days of my cycle. I tried not to think too much of it at the time. My teeth needed some immediate attention though. I knew that those four teeth, the ones missing most of their enamel thanks to my eating disorder, could not be ignored much longer.

When I went to the dentist the verdict was that I had several cavities once again. One tooth had to be pulled, and I needed another root canal. The thinning of my front teeth were definitely a concern to the dentist, so he suggested porcelain crowns. I shared my apprehension about the expense, but he told me I would qualify for coverage because of my mental health history. Despite the terrible health of my teeth, the insurance coverage was good news. I wondered how many more lucky breaks I would be allowed before I had to pay a serious price.

I know that many people get cavities and have root canals, etc., but my teeth were a big psychological trigger for me. They were a constant reminder of my past eating disorder. That was the main reason why I still didn't like going to the dentist. Medically, my abdominal pain also concerned me. I wondered if I had done some irreversible damage. To combat these other physical issues, I was put on an antihypertensive for my high blood pressure and was referred to an OB/GYN for my abdominal pain.

These items may sound trivial to some people and that's okay. Everyone has their "stuff" in life. I guess because I had overcome bulimia and had two difficult labor and deliveries, I hoped that God would lay off for a bit. Medically, I could really use some good news once and a while.

IT'S NOT JUST ME

My sister Kim continued to struggle with her Multiple Sclerosis symptoms. It was around this time that she had her first of four eye surgeries. I don't know where she gets her strength from, but she continues to work fulltime as a medical secretary to this day. I don't think she has too many days where she doesn't feel exhausted, but no matter how tired, Kim is a loving auntie to Ajay and Sammy.

Mick's mom took a downward turn in her prognosis about a year after Sammy was born. She was not doing very well and was in constant pain. Her doctor recommended that she undergo a stem cell transplant, which was a major procedure. They slammed her with chemo after removing all of her teeth because of the extremely high risk of infection. The surgery was very risky, and she stayed in the hospital for about six weeks after the procedure. My father-in-law was there every single day. It was amazing how their roles had changed. She used to do everything for him before she got sick. Now it was his turn to step up to the plate and take care of her ... and he did. The transplant was a success and she did quite well for the next year, almost two. She still took a dozen pills each morning with breakfast and another dozen during the day, but Mick's dad made sure she took them according to doctor's orders. It was actually quite heartwarming to see how much he cared for her.

So despite my issues, I was well aware that many people have personal struggles, both physical and mental. I knew better than to feel sorry for myself as at least my struggles were no longer life-threatening.

THE STRUGGLES OF MENTAL HEALTH

Despite having control over my eating disorder, I still had moments of anxiety and episodes of depression. You may ask what that means exactly. Everyone has times when they feel anxious or are stressed out, right? And we all have times when we are in a gloomier mood than usual, don't we? "So what makes you so different, Andrea?" you may ask. In my opinion, you are right. In some ways I'm not that different. We all experience a variety of emotions day to day, week to week. When we're happy, we laugh. When a loved one dies, we cry. The biggest difference between someone that struggles with a mental illness, like me, and someone that does not is that people with a mental illness tend to get stuck in a depressive mood or cycle of emotion for a much longer period of time than someone who doesn't struggle. Contrarily, someone that is mentally healthy can regulate their emotions and return to a state of homeostasis or "balance" after experiences of high anxiety.

So, for example, do you feel tired, sad, or anxious for an extended period of time, or are you able to level off and feel energetic, happy, or calm once again after a reasonable amount of time? Generally speaking, can your body and mind return to a state of "equilibrium" without much external assistance? My point is simply this. If a negative mood or thought stays with us for a lengthy period of time and it begins to affect the daily activities of living our life, then it is a problem. I'm a psychiatric nurse, so of course I have some background in mental health, but I share my insight more from my personal experiences rather than from what I studied or have seen at work. Many friends and family have heard me joke, "Not only am I the owner, I'm a client." I joked about it, but it was actually true. I studied these topics at school and treated people with mental health issues at work, yet I still struggle with my own mental health disorders. For me, it has always been easier to help someone else with their struggles, than it has been to help myself … but thankfully I'm getting a little better at it with each new day.

Our hectic life often created moments where I felt overwhelmed. Even though I had two healthy kids and a wonderful husband, I would often still feel like I couldn't be a good mom or wife. My psychiatrist would tell me that he didn't understand my self-doubt. I was already doing all of the things that I said I couldn't do. My general practitioner basically told me the same thing. The only area where I felt truly confident, after years of experience, was my job as a psychiatric nurse. I enjoyed helping others, especially with their mental health, and I usually preached what I needed to practice myself. I suspect we can all be guilty of that at times.

SOME PERSONAL ADVICE - SHIFT YOUR MINDSET

I'm going to take a moment and share a few *Do's and Don'ts* that I have learned over the past couple decades through the professional help I received from counsellors and through the team at the BridgePoint Center For Eating Disorders. I'm not sure if these thoughts should be considered "self-help tips", or just caring advice. Either way, I've gathered my thoughts into these eight statements. They deeply resonate with me so I wanted to share them with you as well. I hope they can help you *Shift Your Mindset* much like they helped me shift my thinking:

1. **Avoid letting a single event, somebody's actions, or a statement from others destroy or negatively overwhelm your mood:** I used to really struggle with this personal trait, as I was an emotional sponge. I would soak up any negativism around me and assume it was my fault. Thankfully, I have been able to gradually retrain my thinking. I can now usually differentiate between situations that are within my control and those which are outside of my control. As a result, I have been able to significantly decrease the incidents where my mood is negatively impacted by circumstances outside of my control. If someone is upset about one of life's trivial matters, I now realize that internalizing their frustrations is like a harmful virus for my mental health.

2. **Try not to dwell on the past and stop asking the "why me" questions. See your "failures" as learning opportunities:** I think I can safely say that many of us have "skeletons in our closet" that haunt us. The key is to continue on with your life, moving forward in a positive light, without letting the past overwhelm or inhibit future growth and happiness. Dwelling on the "why me" questions will sap you of the energy needed to heal.

Instead, embrace these moments and trust that the most impactful learning in life most often happens through our mistakes, our misfortunes, and our failures ... so please stop beating yourself up about them.

3. **Stop trying to please everyone else:** I definitely was a hard-core "people pleaser" from a very young age. I realize, to a much lesser degree, that I still have some of these tendencies today. In the past though, almost everything that I did was done with the "feelings of others" in mind ... and instead I suppressed my own feelings. My one selfish act, my eating disorder, was how I manage my emotional stressors. I have learned since, that no matter how hard I try, I cannot make everyone happy. With each new day, I am becoming more and more okay with this reality. So my advice, stop trying to please everyone else and focus on just being yourself. It is a very liberating feeling.

4. **Try not to assume failure or a negative outcome before you even begin. Give yourself a realistic and optimistic chance to succeed:** People often ask, "Is the glass half empty or half full?" In my experience the answer to this question is highly reliant on your mental health. Your state of mind can be a precursor to the outcome. If you have a negative mindset, you are probably doomed to fail. However, with a positive mindset you can accomplish many realistic and amazing personal goals.

5. **Try not to put undue pressure on yourself to be perfect. Nobody is perfect, so it is unfair to assume that you have to be perfect:** I was always very accepting and forgiving of other people's imperfections. However, I certainly did not have that same compassion for myself. I was always my own worst critic. Now I understand that we are all unique individuals and that

we all need to learn to love ourselves just the way we are ...
Imperfections and all.

6. **Try not to make "Mountains out of Molehills":** This tip could
be stated another way too ... such as *"Don't sweat the small stuff!"*
Basically, what I mean is to keep things in perspective. Does
a situation really need all of the attention and emotion you are
investing into it? Often the impact of the external influences
on the rest of your life is not as bad as you think ... so in those
somewhat stressful and frustrating moments, remember that
you are still in control of how you react. Is the world about to
end or is tomorrow just another day? Always try to balance your
emotional-thinking with some logical-thinking to avoid unnecessary overreactions.

7. **Resist the "all or nothing" attitude. There is always a happy
medium:** I think this tip will resonate with most people that
struggle with disordered eating. As a bulimic, I could not just eat
a few cookies. Not because they tasted so good, but because even
when I just ate a few of them it was a symbolism of failure ...
and if I failed, I might as well fail miserably! As a result, I would
eat the whole bag and more. Restriction of food led to overeating
and fueled my vicious cycle of bulimia. This can be true for many
things in life, not just food.

8. **Stop trying so hard to cure yourself. You are not broken
and you are not alone in this fight:** If you have an eating disorder similar to mine, then you need to seek professional help.
You can stop these self-harming behaviours with a little help,
but give yourself the gift of time and forgiveness to heal. Once
you open your mind and heart to outside help you will feel the
heavy burden of "curing yourself" lift off your shoulders. Yes, my
self-reflection and my journaling did help me mend, but I am

certain that I could not have done it alone. Ongoing professional counselling and the intensive inpatient services I received at the BridgePoint Center For Eating Disorders were both keys in my healing. Don't forget that many people struggle with eating disorders and mental illnesses, so you are never alone as long as you are open to help.

I wish I had this insight and knowledge twenty-five years ago. I could have saved myself a significant amount of unnecessary turmoil. Unfortunately, that wasn't the case and my healing journey was a lengthy one as a result. Without a doubt, "stuffing my feelings" as an adolescent was the catalyst for other addictive tendencies such as overeating and purging. Whether you are a parent, teacher, coach, or companion ... please encourage anyone that you suspect to be struggling with their mental health to share their feelings and seek professional help. Expressing our feelings and seeking mental health assistance should not be considered as a sign of weakness by society. Instead we need to view this self-awareness as a positive and necessary step in maintaining or improving our personal health and holistic wellbeing. Slowly and surely, if we are able to increase societal awareness and government funding for mental health, a day will come when nobody has to feel ashamed anymore. Just as there is no shame in "getting cancer", much like my mother-in-law, there should be no embarrassment in "being mentally ill" ... but unfortunately, many of our family, friends, and neighbours are still hiding in the shadows of ridicule and perceived weakness.

If we normalize mental illnesses, much like any physical ailment, then hopefully those that suffer will seek professional help sooner in their lives. As we work together to lift the stigmas surround mental health, we also need to lobby for increased mental health funding. As we know, these illnesses do not play favourites, nor do they only impact a specific gender, age, or ethnicity. There is a real good chance that a disorder has impacted your life, or someone very special to you.

Coming forward for help is only half of the equation, the other half is ensuring that the necessary resources are available to treat the ill. Currently, adequate funding for mental health facilities and other proactive interventions, especially in the area of disordered eating, is severely lacking. Early intervention programs in schools, alongside recovery programs such as the BridgePoint Center For Eating Disorders, could prevent addictive habits from becoming engrained in our youth … and help them, as in my case, avoid sixteen years of hell.

LIFE JUST KEEPS ROLLING ALONG

Fast forward to a scheduled hysterectomy surgery. My uterus had continued to spasm on a monthly basis, and the pain was often intense. The only solution was surgery. The procedure went well and my OB/GYN discovered that I also had endometriosis, so the surgery was a necessity.

Career-wise, I decided it was best to take a job at Langenburg's Centennial Special Care Home, a long-term care facility. Even though I enjoyed my job on the psychiatric Pine Unit in Yorkton, the driving back and forth each day was getting tiresome. As a result, I also resigned from the Churchbridge Public School, which I would dearly miss, but the part-time hours could not financially compete with the new opportunity. The care home position would challenge me in a new way, as I would need to brush up on a few medical skills that I hadn't used for several years. It turned out to be a good move, as I discovered a joy for working at the care home as well. We are like a big family there, and I have many wonderful colleagues, but the most rewarding part of the job for me was simply talking with the residents and comforting them.

So much happened in the next eight or so years, but I won't bore you with all of it. My husband was now the principal of the high school. It was a very busy job, definitely not a Monday-Friday and nine o'clock to three-thirty job like many people think it is. Mick's mom was slowly deteriorating. We made at least four emergency trips to Calgary, on top of our regular visits to see them, because doctors called to say that she didn't have long to live. Without a doubt, it was an emotional roller coaster ride. However, for many years, no matter how badly her health deteriorated she kept fighting. Severe pneumonia, H1N1, and many other fatal diagnoses were no match for her, as she always found a way to pull through with the help of her doctors and husband. I admired her toughness. Not only her physical toughness, but her emotional and mental toughness too. The continual stream of medical bad news would have emotionally devastated many people, but instead it just seemed to motivate her to fight even harder. She said she wasn't ready to give up quite yet as there was too much to live for, especially all her grandchildren.

One visit to Calgary, in particular, is worth mentioning in more detail. My father-in-law's health had also been deteriorating over the years. His daily walks had pretty much all but come to a halt because of his shortness of breath. In his late-fifties, he had open heart surgery (a quintuple bypass). Now at the age of seventy-four, he needed to get a pacemaker and defibrillator inserted in his chest to help regulate his heart rate. The surgeon said he would need to stay in the hospital for a few days. We decided this was a good time to make a visit.

Mommy was doing about the same as the last time we visited. I was in constant awe of how she kept going. She was slow-moving, but she still got around the house pretty well using her walker. I instantly noticed a difference in Daddy though. He had lost a significant amount of weight, and the energy was missing in his gait. This was a big change from the fellow who took brisk daily walks through the city parks and to the grocery store just a few months ago. When asked about it, Daddy didn't like to focus on his own health. He was only worried about his wife's health and said he would go back for a checkup with his doctor once Mommy was feeling better.

Daddy's shortness of breath was very evident, even when he just walked up the stairs from the basement in their bungalow condo. On the second last day of our visit, Mick took his mom to her appointment at the Tom Baker Cancer Centre. They left around six in the morning and were gone most of the day. After breakfast, the boys went downstairs to play. Daddy said he was going to have a nap as he was feeling tired, but instead he sat down on the couch and started chatting with me. He was short of breath even after speaking only a few short sentences. I encouraged him to take his nitro spray, but his answer always was that he didn't want to get "addicted" to it. That made me giggle as he was quite paranoid about the medication. I told him to trust Nurse Andrea and to not worry about getting addicted. I could tell that he respected my advice.

Our conversation continued, but this time it was not like the "other talks" we've had in the past. Usually, he would tell me about growing up in his village in India, working in England, and the sacrifices it took to move Mommy and Mick's older siblings, Harprit and Jodie, to Canada in 1965 ... Mick wasn't born until a couple years later at the Regina General Hospital. This time, however, the conversation focused more on his feelings about family. He said he was proud of "Minky", which was Mick's childhood nickname, and was proud of all his children. He then asked me to make sure that Mick knew that he admired how Mick had turned out to be a successful teacher, a caring husband, and a loving father. I teased him that he should tell Mick himself, but in the end I promised to share his thoughts. Daddy also shared that he thought of me as his daughter, that they were lucky to have me as part of their family, and that Mick was blessed to have me as his wife. That almost brought tears to my eyes. The strangest part of our chat was that he kept saying that he should "go lay down now" about every half hour. Instead we talked for hours. He would proceed to his bedroom, but then turn around. He would come back sit on the couch and start talking to me again about family. I soon found out why he wanted to keep talking.

Mick returned with his mom later that afternoon, and she went to lay down as she was exhausted from her long day of tests at the hospital. Daddy was finally napping too. I told Mick about the lengthy conversation I had with his dad. I expressed that I found it a bit odd that his dad just wanted to keep talking about how proud he was of all his family, despite being so tired, weak, and short of breath. Even though I was flattered by his sincere compliments, I was concerned that there was more going on than what Daddy led onto.

We left Calgary the next day as planned, with Daddy promising he would go see his doctor later that week. We drove to Regina and spent the night at my parents' house. Mick's mom and dad always reminded us to call when we arrived to our destination. I gave them a quick call from Regina as it was getting late, and told them I would call again when we got back to Langenburg.

The next day, when we got home, I unpacked while Mick shovelled the driveway. After supper, Mick and some friends decided to get together to play some cards. I called Calgary around 8:00 p.m. and Daddy answered the phone. He was happy to hear that we made it home, but his voice sounded very weak. He said good-bye more quickly than usual, and handed the phone to Mommy. She immediately started crying. "Oh Andrea, he is not doing well. I am scared." She continued on, but I can't remember her exact words. I asked if she had phoned her older son Jodie, as he now lived in Calgary too. She had tried calling Jodie but there was no answer. I reassured her that Daddy would be okay even though I wasn't too sure of that myself. This wasn't the first time that she had voiced her concerns about Daddy's health to me, so I said, "Make sure you tell him to rest and take his nitro spray. I will tell Mick to call you back."

I called Mick on his cell phone and eventually got through to him around nine o'clock. "You better call your mom. She's pretty worked up about your dad," I said. Mick assured me he would call, so I went to bed. Mick came home around 11:00 p.m. with a couple friends that were unusually quiet. I could tell Mick was upset. He said, "I think my dad is dying," as he broke into tears. "I have been on the phone for the last couple hours talking with doctors and things really don't sound good. I couldn't get a hold of Jodie, so I called 911 in Calgary to get an ambulance for my dad. My aunt went over to the house, but Mom is pretty upset." This was the first time Mick openly sobbed in front of his friends, so I knew he was devastated too.

We spent most of the night on the phone, but were finally told by the nurses that we should just get some sleep and they would update us in the morning ... unfortunately, Daddy didn't make it until the morning. At around 6:30 a.m. we got a call stating that he wasn't able to recover from the heart attack that he had the previous evening. The date was February 27, 2012 ... R.I.P. Daddy ... we miss you.

TRYING TO HELP PICK UP THE PIECES

A few hours later, we were on the road back to Calgary, a quick 48-hour turnaround. We got there about suppertime, and the house was already filled with mourning relatives. Mommy sat on the couch in an almost comatose state. She cried so hard when we hugged her. You could tell she lost her "one and only". As part of cultural tradition, the living room floor was covered with white sheets and most of the people were sitting on the floor. It was Monday and the funeral wasn't till Saturday, so much of the week was spent visiting with relatives and other family friends who came over to pay their respects and to mourn. I soon figured out that the best way I could help out was to make the Chai tea and serve it to our visitors. Mick's younger brother, Sterling, and his family arrived from Surrey, B.C. later that day. Mick's sister, Harprit, and her boys would come later in the week from British Columbia as well.

The three brothers, Jodie, Sterling, and Mick had a busy week completing funeral arrangements. Each day Mommy just sat or laid on the couch moaning and crying. There was an average of at least fifty people visiting per day all week long ... so many people. I had no idea that Daddy was so well known and respected in Calgary. My parents drove in from Regina and stayed at my aunt and uncle's house about thirty minutes away. They stopped by the house to say hello to Mick's mom, Rajinder, but understandably she was not overly talkative as she was exhausted from all the previous visitors.

I worried about Rajinder. I knew the steady traffic through the house would take a toll on her body due to her weakened immune system. As I suspected, on Wednesday morning when I went to check on her in the bedroom, she sounded awful. I suspected the issue was pneumonia, which she had had about ten times since her initial cancer diagnosis. With all the people she was around this week, her chances of getting sick dramatically increased. My sister-in-law, also a nurse, agreed that Mommy needed to go to the hospital. With much persuasion, Rajinder finally agreed to let us call the ambulance.

The hospital admitted her with double pneumonia. Her oxygen levels were very low. She definitely needed to be there or she would have only gotten worse. My heart went out to her. The poor lady was trying to deal with her husband's death, and now she was deathly ill herself. The doctor wanted to keep her in the hospital for at least a week. Mick discussed the upcoming funeral with the doctor. The physician said he would evaluate whether she was well enough to attend the funeral in a few days ... the possibility of not being able to attend your spouse's funeral seemed almost cruel.

Back at the house, the amount of people dropping by slowed down now that Mommy was in the hospital. Harprit and her boys had arrived. Everything was pretty much in order for Saturday's funeral except for Mommy's health. It wasn't until the day before the funeral that the doctor informed us that he would grant a day pass from the hospital. He was very concerned about her compromised immune system, but he knew he could not deny her wish. Not being able to attend would have been devastating and maybe even worse.

Mick picked up his mom for the funeral the next day. She was still quite lethargic, but very glad that she could attend. Mick gave a heartfelt eulogy. People laughed and people cried. Mick even said a few words in his hilarious "Bollywood" accent, which always made his dad laugh. Rajinder giggled too as she knew Mick always did the accent to tease his dad, similarly to how comedian Russell Peters made fun of his own dad during his hilarious shows.

A few hours after the funeral, Mick took Rajinder back to the hospital. She was exhausted again, but at peace with being able to experience the ceremony. It was another week until she was strong enough to come home. Jodie and his boys moved in with Mommy to help care for her. She definitely could not live on her own, plus she could really use the company of her grandchildren to fill her new void. I wondered how she would do without her husband. He had done so much for her since she had gotten sick, so I feared her sadness would take its toll.

ON A ROLL ... BUT NOT A GOOD ONE

Tarsem's death, was the first of three tragedies to happen within eighteen months. As many people say, "Bad things often happen in life in three's," and unfortunately they did for us too.

For the most part, life went back to normal for us in Langenburg. We called Mommy on a regular basis to check in and let her know that we were thinking of her. Our nephews, Jodie's boys, were really good with their grandma and she loved having them there. Despite the company, she still missed her husband. Christmas was nearing once again so we made plans to go to Calgary. Rajinder said she was looking forward to seeing us. I still often thought of Mick's dad and felt honored by the way he shared his final thoughts with me. The visits to Calgary would definitely feel different without him there.

It was around the first week in December when I called Mommy for one of our weekly chats. She was having constant physical pain, but I think some of it may have also been the pain of a broken heart. Over the past few months she even made some comments about "joining" her husband. I tried to encourage her and convince her that she still had so much to live for. I reassured her that we would be seeing her soon and that we would have a fun visit.

On December 17th at about 11:00 p.m. Mick got a call from his older brother. Jodie called an ambulance to take Mommy to the hospital. He had her at the doctor a few days prior and she was on oral antibiotics for a mild case of pneumonia, but the medication obviously wasn't working. Even though we always worried, we didn't start to panic because contracting pneumonia had become very common for her over the past five years. In addition, Jodie was with her and Rajinder was always so tough. We hoped that she would be fine after some medical attention. Jodie promised to keep us posted.

Very early the next morning, Jodie called and said that Mommy was in an induced coma. The infection had spread throughout her entire body, which is called sepsis. He sent us a picture of her. Mick and I now started to panic. The picture showed her laying in an intensive care hospital bed with tubes and wires all over her body. I chatted with another nurse-friend who had some experience with this sort of patient condition, and she said to start preparing for the worst. A little later that day, Jodie called with an update. Doctors told him there was zero chance that Mommy would recover. Her body had shut down, and she would not survive this time. Mommy passed away on December 18, 2012, only ten months after her husband left her ... R.I.P. Mommy ... I will miss our talks on the phone and our giggles while we watched our afternoon television soap operas together.

Our kids were very sad. They had lost Calgary Papa and now Calgary Grammy in such a short timeframe. I cried with them when Mick told the boys the sad news. Sammy was seven and a half years old and Ajay would be nine years old in January, so both old enough to have a close connection with their grandparents. I'll never forget what Sammy said after Mick told him about Grammy, "It will be okay Daddy, because Grammy is with Papa in heaven now and she doesn't have to feel sad anymore." That sure made a lot of sense to me.

TAKE TWO

We were off to Calgary the next morning. Mick and Jodie were responsible for making the funeral arrangements once again. I remember feeling really sad for Jodie's three boys. They had lost their mom to cancer when they were five, six, and thirteen years old respectively. Then they moved from Toronto to Calgary and were living with Calgary Grammy when she passed away. So they had lost their mom, their grandpa, and now grandma. I knew how sad Ajay and Sammy felt, so I could only imagine how Jodie's boys felt after losing so many important family members in their short lives.

We arrived in Calgary, and it felt like a bad dream that was repeating itself. The only difference this time was that it was mostly relatives and close friends that stopped by the house, and not the whole cultural community. I think that was partly because Mommy had been battling cancer for nine long years so her passing was not as unexpected as Daddy's death. Also, since Mick and his siblings never grew up in Calgary, they only had ties with relatives and not the entire community like their parents. It was, however, nice to see the aunties, uncles and cousins. They were always so caring and generous. Many of them were tearful, of course, but they were also relieved that

Mommy's long and painful battle with cancer was finally over. She had suffered so much, constantly in and out of hospitals and rehab facilities. We were fortunate to have her around as long as we did considering that doctors only gave her six to twelve months to live when she was first diagnosed with cancer. Instead, because she battled for eight additional years, she got to see, hold, and play with all nine of her grandchildren. Unfortunately, her quality of life only got worse once Daddy passed away. As a result, Mick sadly got to share two eulogies in less than a year.

We arrived back in Langenburg just before the New Year. It felt strange not having to call Calgary when we arrived safely. I thought of all of our trips to Calgary over the past twelve years. Honestly, I can say that deep down, I too was relieved that Mommy wasn't suffering anymore. I guess her prayers from her last few months had been answered. I often thought of Tarsem and Rajinder, and what Sammy said about them being together again. That brought a smile to my face and some peace to my heart because Sammy was right ... that is exactly what Grammy wanted most, to be with Papa.

A DEVASTATING SUMMER

The year 2013 started out fine considering the hurt of 2012. We kept busy with work and the boys' sports. I was having issues with my lower back, on and off for the past two years, but I managed to continue working. After all we had been through lately, I was determined to "suck it up" because things could always be worse. As always, Mick was busy with one new challenge after another at work. The province, the school division, and the community were in the early planning stages of building a brand new school in Langenburg due to air quality issues in the current high school. The new facility was to be completed by the fall of 2016, so Mick had to attend many planning meetings that year.

Before we knew it, summer was here and we were excited about our plans to go back to Columbia Falls, Montana with my immediate family. We planned to stay at my parents' timeshare, located on a beautiful golf course. The golfers in our family loved that, plus it was surrounded by mountains, gorgeous lakes, and the beaches of the scenic Whitefish area. Most of the Gilbert (a.k.a. Griswold's as nicknamed by Mick) family was going, so it was going to be fun ... just what the doctor ordered after such a difficult year. Mick and I were looking so forward to spending some quality time with the boys and my family.

We spent the night before leaving for Montana in Regina. For the most part, we were packed and ready to hit the "holiday road" bright and early the next morning. Ajay and Sammy were really excited because the last time we were in Montana was two years ago. They were only seven and six then, but they remembered bits and pieces of the last trip, so they knew that they were going to have fun playing watersports with their cousins. My brother and his family arrived at my parents' house, and Mick was packing the last suitcase into our car. My mom and I had just finished making some sandwiches and were filling the cooler with snacks. We were just about ready to get on the road.

A few minutes later Mick came back into the house and instead of saying, "Come on, let's get going," like he often does when he is eager to hit the road, he just stood quietly by the door. I will never forget the look I saw on his face. It was like he had just seen a ghost. He continued to stand in the entryway and stare at the cell phone in his hand. "Honey," I asked, "What's the matter?" He didn't answer right away and just kept staring at his phone. "Mick, what's wrong? You are starting to scare me," I asked again. He finally responded. "My younger brother Sterling, he's gone." I was completely dumbfounded and asked him to clarify, "What do you mean he's gone?" By the devastation on Mick's face, I soon figured out what he meant. So very sadly, Mick's thirty-nine-year-old brother died while playing in a recreational ice hockey game. A few first responders that happened to be playing in the same hockey game tried to revive him using a defibrillator without success.

The pain I felt for my husband and his extended family was surreal. "What the hell is happening to my family?" Mick said with a sense of shock. I think he hoped it was some kind of bad dream. It was his older brother, Jodie, who had called with the devastating news. My whole family was at a loss for words. My mom hugged Mick. The rest of my family offered their condolences as well. Mick went upstairs into the bedroom and sat on the bed. I hugged him so hard while tears poured down my face. He just sat quietly for a few minutes and then said, "We need to leave for B.C. right now." We decided that we would drive to Calgary today, spend the night with Jodie, and then continue on to Surrey, British Columbia tomorrow morning.

For the third time in eighteen months, Ajay and Sammy were sad for their dad. Once again, they were old enough to understand the seriousness of what just happened. Even though they were looking forward to having fun in Montana with their cousins, they were so very understanding and considerate of why our plans had to change. They too were very saddened that Uncle Sterling had passed away. The date was July 12, 2013 ... R.I.P. Sterling.

The next week felt like a repetitive bad dream, but as Mick said, "It is one thing to lose your parents, especially if you know they are ill, but it's another thing to lose a healthy younger brother ... it's just not right." It was a very difficult funeral. We felt so badly for Sterling's wife, and of course his children, his young son and beautiful little daughter ... they were his pride and joy ... it was such a tragedy.

We arrived back in Langenburg about two weeks later. Some of our friends put together a big basket filled with many thoughtful condolence gifts. We were touched and so appreciative. Our lawn was nicely cut and my flowers had been watered. We had so many wonderful friends and were very grateful for what we still had ... each other, our extended families, and our close friends. I also reminded myself of the Serenity Prayer … It once again gave me a sense of comfort and peace amidst the chaos of life.

SOME NEW LIFE HURDLES

Physically, I had several struggles. My chronic back pain, from a previous injury, continued to get worse. At times, I couldn't work. Recently, I also began experiencing frequent muscle twitches, balance problems, sore hands, leg cramps, and a few other symptoms. At one point I was told by a doctor that I most likely had Raynaud's Syndrome because I often had cold hands and feet, which also frequently got numb for a short periods of time. Fibromyalgia was also a possibility based on my symptoms. Either way, I kept plugging away at work and accepted that these symptoms were not that serious. However, as time lapsed, my symptoms seemed to get worse and worse. I started to doubt that the problems were minor. I wondered if my doctors, just like Mommy's original doctor, thought that I was imagining some of these symptoms. Mick tried to make light of the situation by joking that I should get a frequent-user discount with the doctors, as I seemed to have another medical appointment every month. Although we both tried to find some humor to combat my physical pain, the symptoms were becoming more troublesome with each passing year.

On February 16, 2016, I was diagnosed with Multiple Sclerosis. A few months earlier my general practitioner referred me to the neurologist once again. A new MRI of my brain and of my spinal cord were ordered due to the increased muscle and nerve pain. Unfortunately, compared to the MRI taken five years ago, this new MRI confirmed that I had a significant increase in the amount and size of the lesions in my brain and spinal cord. This was typical evidence that neurologists used to diagnose patients with Multiple Sclerosis.

Honestly, I did not take the news very well. What next? Wasn't it enough that I struggled with an eating disorder for years and now this? I was upset and Mick was trying to be strong for the both of us. Mick said, "We will get through this one together too." I love him so much. Later, Mick gathered the boys and told them about Mommy's disease. It was the same disease that their Auntie Kim was struggling with for the past twenty-three years, so they were somewhat familiar with what MS can do to a person. "Sometimes, it can make your balance a little funny and hurt your eyes, like Auntie Kim's eye," they said. Kim, being the wonderful sister that she is, reassured me that she would be there for me too, even if it was just to vent.

My parents had just left for Arizona the previous day ... what is with the Griswold vacations? Something bizarre always seems to happen every time they plan a getaway! I decided that I did not want to tell them my bad news while they were on vacation, as they needed a break from life too. However, since my mom knew I had a specialist appointment with the neurologist, she pried the truth out of me over the phone. Now she had two daughters with MS, and I had a whole new set of life hurdles to deal with.

MY NEW REALITY

The emotions that I felt on the day that I was diagnosed with Multiple Sclerosis were complex. Naturally, I felt devastated by the diagnosis, but in another way I felt somewhat validated. Let me explain that.

The physical symptoms that I was experiencing were nothing new. I had been living with them for years, they were just gradually worsening. In the past, I was told that the tingling in my feet could be attributed to sciatica and at worst the tightness in my legs may be due to a mild form of Fibromyalgia. I felt that my physical pain was worsening, but when my specialists hadn't found any definite medical issues related to the pain previously, I did begin to think that maybe I was imagining these symptoms … maybe they were the result of just "another one of Andrea's mental health disorders". I was consumed by self-doubt. Was I sick or was I just "depressed or going crazy"… or maybe it was a little of both?

My concerns heightened once my vision started to get blurry. I also found that when I got tired, my face started to occasionally go numb and droop, which would sometimes slur my speech. That's when I decided to let my general practitioner know what was going on, and he decided to refer me to the neurologist. It was the same neurologist I had seen initially about my back pain and my sciatica issues. On the visit five years previous, I was exposed to a full body MRI where they "accidentally" found lesions in my brain. That was followed up with a spinal tap to test for auto-immune diseases. However, because the spinal tap did not indicate any auto-immune disease, the specialist concluded that the symptoms were most likely due to the moderate disc degeneration in my L5-S1 and possibly also due to sciatica flare-ups. I was relieved with this news, however, part of me began to feel like my doctors, family, and friends were beginning to dismiss my physical complaints … and perhaps I was "imagining" them? Either way, I was definitely dealing with a medical issue, whether it was physical, mental, or both.

Ironically, finally confirmed five years later by the increased lesions in my brain, I now have some sense of validation. At least I can now say that it's not "all in my head" … and I am not just imagining these symptoms … the source of the discomfort is very real. Yay! Congratulations Andrea. Do I win a prize? Of course, in reality I would have loved to be wrong and not feel any discomfort. So despite the chance of others finding it odd, knowing that I'm not imagining these symptoms is a bizarre form of consolation for me.

The neurologist immediately ordered five days of intravenous steroids to shrink the lesions and calm my symptoms. I began the treatments as soon as we returned home to Langenburg. We made five trips to the Esterhazy Hospital and each treatment took about an hour and a half. I was warned that I would feel worse before I felt better because the medication is usually pretty hard on the patients system, and that is exactly what is happening. It's been a few days now since my final intravenous dose, but I don't think I can write too much more today because I am exhausted ... time to take a break.

WHO KNOWS WHAT LIES AHEAD?

My husband has been through so much with me, and I am so grateful that he hasn't given up on me. My boys are the greatest kids I could ever ask for. I also can't forget about our puppy Jazzie, who had been with our family for almost sixteen years (She passed away two weeks after I was diagnosed with MS). If it was possible, I'm sure Jazzie would have had plenty of stories to share ... she had seen it all, the good times, the bad times, and the really dark times. My parents and my siblings have also always been there for me. I am very appreciative that we have such a close-knit family. I also have the best friends in the world. My dining room table is full of flowers, and my fridge is full of food thanks to my friends. I feel very blessed despite this new personal hurdle that I must find a way over.

Even with all of my flaring aches and pains, in some ways I feel more determined to make a difference in the lives of young girls, boys, and adults who struggle with bulimia and other eating disorders. I feel as if God has put me to the challenge. He may put additional hurdles in my path, perhaps even bigger than overcoming an eating disorder, but I truly think that He wants me to do something with all of the knowledge I have gained from these turmoil-filled experiences in my life. One thing I am certain of is that I was born to help people … I have just been waiting for some direction on a meaningful purpose and cause. I think that I have now found it.

So, I say to myself at the top of my lungs, "Bring it on, God. I am ready for the challenge, and I promise to try and make a small difference in this world before my time on it is up. If my motivation and my ability to help others is due to my experience of living with a mental illness and through my years of battling with an eating disorder, then I must thank you, God." I refuse to say that I wish it all never happened and that I wish I could change my past, as I would not be who I am today … a mother of two beautiful boys, a spouse to a wonderful man, a psychiatric nurse who gets to care for those with mental illnesses, but most importantly, I can now look in the mirror and be happy with who I am. So, I will only move forward, not backwards, and I will use my past to make a positive change in the world.

I believe we all have personal challenges and difficult choices to make. I could easily fade away and just feel sorry for myself, because of my recent Multiple Sclerosis diagnosis. I refuse. Even if my efforts only help a single individual climb out of their dark hole, it will be worth it. Therefore, I hope that the past fourteen years of pouring out the ugly truth of my eating disorder on paper will somehow connect with those in need and help them the way it has helped me. So please remember, no matter what mental, physical, or emotional struggle you are currently battling, that you are never alone even if it may often feel like it. There are people who care about you and that want to help you. Remember that things will get better as long as you do not give up on yourself. And most importantly, always remember that you are worth it.

THE FINAL CHAPTER

Today is October 20, 2016. I am on my second trial of MS medication, as the first attempt to curb my symptoms did not work very well. Many of the trial drugs currently have harsh side effects and can actually do more harm than good for some individuals, so my neurologist is constantly monitoring my overall health. I am hoping this new medication will help relieve some of the symptoms as they seem to be worsening. I miss being at work, but I have accepted where I am at physically. I know that some of the physical responsibilities of being a nurse at the care home would be challenging. I hope that someday soon, I will be able to return to work and help patients with their emotional and mental hurdles. Honestly, being off work has been a real tough pill to swallow. I suppose, just like everyone else that is managing physical and/or mental health issues, I can only do the best I can … one day at a time.

When I started writing this journal many years ago, I really didn't expect to continue the reflective process for very long, let alone follow it through to completion. I realize now that this was an unattainable goal, because this healing process does not have a definitive finish line for me; it will continue to be a work in progress and evolve. This writing process didn't feel like a "work project" either, because I was in control of how far I took it. I didn't have any deadlines to meet and, initially at least, I was just doing it for myself. The only person I had to answer to was me. Maybe that's why it has taken so long for me to share my story. Yet, this commitment to reflective therapy has been like no other prior experience. The emotional and physiological reactions that I felt when I went back to those dark moments were sometimes overwhelming, but healing as well. I learned to be very honest with myself and I learned to stop being ashamed of my past. There is no denying who I was, and there is no shame in who I have become as a result. So, you may ask if all the time and effort I put into journaling was worth it. Without a doubt, my overwhelming answer is "Yes". I would encourage anyone who is struggling with a mental illness to give journaling a try. If you stick with it, it can be an incredible healing process when paired with mental health intervention and ongoing professional counselling services.

WHAT'S THE POINT ANDREA?

So was this book supposed to be about eating disorders, or life in general? Good question ... at times I'm not even sure myself. If I had completed this writing process before our family tragedies and my MS diagnosis, then I'm certain that my sole focus would have been on bulimia and addictions. However, I believe every significant event in our life changes our direction ... and who we are, even if we do not recognize the change in the moment. If I had written only about my eating disorder experiences, then these words would not tell my complete story. I want people to know that, "Yes, sometimes life sucks." However, you are never alone. So, find the courage to fight and get the help you need to live a better life. Nobody else can or will do it for you. I now realize that we all have challenges and that we all are products of our past experiences. In the past, my perception was that everyone else was stronger than me because they were able to bounce back from their life struggles on their own, but for some reason I could not. I was also too stubborn to admit that I had a problem or that I needed help. I now realize, that needing support is nothing to be ashamed about. Whether it is physical help, emotional help, or psychological help ... everyone will need a helping hand sometime in their life. So, whatever your story is, don't feel ashamed to seek out support.

Also realize that you are not at the mercy of destiny. You can impact change. You can be in control of your decisions and your life. You just may need a little push getting there. Thankfully, many people in my life inspired me to change, otherwise I still might be stuck in a vicious eating disorder cycle to this day. I admire the "get up, dust yourself off, and go try again" attitude that many people possess. There was a time that I didn't possess any of those qualities, but now I am getting closer and closer to being that strong. With each passing day, I am more confident that I will someday be strong enough and wise enough to help others that are stuck in the destructive cycle of an eating disorder. As a matter of fact, I just happen to know a few things about the topic ... you may say, that I'm somewhat of a self-taught expert!

This may also shock you (yes, I mean it sarcastically), but like most couples, my marriage is not perfect either ... and what does a perfect marriage look like anyways? I have often said to Mick that I think most couples would have "packed it in by now" if they had to live our marriage. We have been through many struggles together. Mostly my stuff, but stuff from his side of the family as well. Yet, here we are, still together and still looking out for each other. I'm not sure if it is due more to love or to loyalty, but thankfully we found a way to survive it all. And yes, I acknowledge that many couples have been through highly stressful marital hardships, even much worse than our experiences, and they have found a way to flourish as a couple. I believe the secret to a happy marriage is to focus on the people in your life, your partner and your kids, and not on the day to day turmoil that may surround you. There will always be something to complain about. Enjoy the company of the people in your life and remember that laughter is always the best medicine.

So, despite my newest hurdle of Multiple Sclerosis, my focus will continue to be on trying to create positive change in this world. I will share my life-learnings, through the eyes of a bulimic, even though I'm sure my MS will continue to present challenges along the way. Do I think my new diagnosis will change my perspective on life? How can it not? As I said before, we are always evolving and life events will continue to leave their fingerprints on my story. As the journey continues,

I will learn to adjust to life with MS and not let it dictate who I am. Therefore, even though I was very devastated upon my initial diagnosis, I now realize this is just one more hurdle that I need to manage, so that I can be there for my kids, my husband, my family, my friends, and most importantly, myself. I've recently learned that overcoming a major hurdle in life, bulimia in my case, doesn't mean that our struggles are over. The accomplishment simply prepares you to be a little stronger and smarter for the next challenge coming your way.

TRY

To not know, is fear
To know, is fear
To not try, is scary
To try, is scary

We do not want to live this way
With emotions overwhelming
We struggle to find the answers
But the "what if's" keep us stuck

Not wanting to fail, or disappoint
We hesitate to ask for help
Until we realize, we do not fail
As long as we just keep trying

JUMPING HURDLES –
THE RACE THAT NEVER ENDS

To me, that is what life is about ... jumping hurdles ... and these hurdles aren't in a straight line like in a track and field race, but instead the race course is really messy and unorganized. Some of the hurdles may be small, so they don't require much work, but others are really big and despite our best efforts it's going take a few attempts to get over them. We will stumble often, and we will get hurt occasionally. We may even shed some tears. It may take us a while to try again because everything inside of us says that we should just give up and quit the fight. Sometimes we need the help of others to get over our injuries, but other times we just need time to mend on our own. It usually helps to have someone to talk to about our feelings of defeat, but self-reflection and meditation can be powerful tools as well. After time, once rested and cared for, we are ready to try again. We stare up at that hurdle that knocked us down previously and for some reason it does not look as high or as intimidating as before. We feel a bit more confident now, maybe just because things are a bit more familiar, and we've learned from our mistakes. We make it over the hurdle, and we feel so good. And rightfully so, we celebrate our success.

But as life would have it, and usually not long after, we encounter another hurdle. This one may seem even bigger than the last one. The negative thinking takes over again, and we don't even want to attempt it this time in fear of failure. We beat ourselves up and feel defeated once again. If we are fortunate, our family and friends gather around us as supports. They say good things about us to make us feel better, but we don't accept the praise because the "tapes" playing in our head convince us otherwise, "You don't deserve to be happy. You are such a loser. You'll never be a good mother."

We often stay stuck and dwell in this type of thinking for days, weeks, months, or even years. Meanwhile, we see friends jumping over their hurdles with ease. We wonder, "Why is it always so hard for me?" We question our self-worth and dabble in self-pity. It may take us awhile, but it's usually in a place we call "rock bottom" that we realize that we must get by this overwhelming hurdle before it's too late. No one else can do it for us. It will require some difficult and emotional work to build up our self-esteem, but ultimately it's our choice to make. Either we continue to fall deeper into our pool of demons, or we begin to climb out. Two steps forward, and one back ... but slowly and surely, we gain the confidence that we can do it.

A few years ago a friend reminded me of an inspirational, but fairly common saying that resonated with me, so here is a version that sums up my life experience ... ***"Pain in life is inevitable, but misery and self-pity in life is optional. You can either be Bitter or you can be Better ... the choice is yours to make.*** Despite the possible over-use of the phrase "Bitter or Better" by therapists and psychiatrists, I still connected with the message. As a result, I wrote the following "Bitter or Better" poem which reflects on my journey to a healthier life and the support of my friends along the way.

BITTER OR BETTER

Sometimes things happen in our life
That do not always go our way
We get angry and start to curse
And these dark feelings tend to stay

Why me God? We start to ask
Life seems so cruel and unfair
The misfortunes are hard to accept
And the weight is too much to bear

Our mood dips and our thinking changes
We've become someone that we do not know
Now when we take a look in the mirror
We're ashamed, as the old self does not show

The world does not seem to understand
And sometimes people don't even care
You become bitter about everything
And friends notice you've lost your flair

Days leave you feeling exhausted
So you just want to run and hide
Then a very good friend shows up
You trust her enough to confide

After some time spent with this good friend
You realize you have a choice to make
It's choosing better, instead of bitter
She's helped you figure out what's at stake

Overcoming bulimia was definitely the biggest hurdle I have ever encountered up until now. Over fifteen years of "get up and try again" is a long time, but I look at my boys today and think, "Thank God I did not give up." There is so much to live for no matter how bad things may get. And, of course, life continues on no matter what, so why not try to enjoy it. Just like everyone else, I will have to keep running and jumping over new obstacles as they present themselves ... and maybe that's why they call us the human race.

MY HUSBAND

I don't know how to thank all the wonderful people in my life who have stuck by me, but I do know who to start with: my husband Mick. He has been through the darkest days with me and helped me stay focused on the light of a better day. Sometimes when a loved one is sick, so much focus and energy is spent dealing with a partner's illness that it can create an enormous amount of stress. I know this journey hasn't been an easy one for Mick. He has always put my needs and our kids' needs before his own.

I also recognize that Mick had his own unique set of emotions, perspectives, and experiences during my most challenging years. So a word of caution to readers, despite my husband's incredible emotional and mental resilience, your partner needs to be mindful of their own mental health. I assume having a life partner, a friend, or a child with an eating disorder would be an exhausting experience. So, even though I try to put myself in Mick's shoes, I can only imagine how distraught he was at times. Communication, open and honest, is the key to staying attached and grounded with each other. However, without a doubt, this is often very difficult to accomplish when one person in the relationship is mentally ill.

Since an eating disorder can put an extraordinary amount of stress on a marriage, Mick and I both felt it was important for him to share a "Partner's Perspective" in this memoir as well. In the following pages, Mick has agreed to briefly share his personal experience of living with a bulimic and what he learned along the way. Since we can rarely walk the bumpy road to recovery alone, our hope is that our story can inspire a sense of optimism and strengthen your faith in each other. Do not be mistaken though, *evolving this hope into action* is where your hard work really begins. I'd like to think that it is never too late to start your healing journey together, but the reality is that some relationships do get damaged beyond repair. Therefore, I encourage couples, family members, and individuals to seek professional help as soon as possible. The dark hole of disordered eating and addiction plays no favorites ... and your relationships are not immune to this disease.

A HUSBAND'S OR A PARTNER'S PERSPECTIVE

Andrea's disordered eating story became a significant chapter in my life story once we were engaged to be married on September 17, 2000 ... my birthday. Our marriage and relationship has truly been a roller coaster ride ever since. The moment I met Andrea, I was drawn to her. Not only was she very pretty, funny, and full of energy, but I recall seeing so much kindness in her eyes. Besides all that, we both loved to dance and laugh together. It felt like we were two pieces of a jigsaw puzzle that were meant to fit together. Yes, I know it sounds cliché, but I do believe "we fell in love" with each other. However, that connection was soon put to the test after I truly realized how strongly addicted Andrea was to her bulimic habits.

Initially, I only had a vague understanding of bulimia. I knew it involved throwing up after eating, but I certainly did not know the real reason why people are bulimic. I simply assumed it was because they didn't want to gain weight. Even though I was partially right, I had no idea how powerful and destructive the addiction could be in someone's life. I didn't have a clue that a bulimic experiences an addictive "high" during their binge. I also didn't know that there was a lot of guilt, shame, self-doubt, and self-harm involved in the purge. I was also unaware that bulimia was a mental health issue, and that the addiction had taken complete control of my fiancée's life. I had no idea that a bulimic lifestyle was Andrea's "normal" and now that we were getting married, that bulimia would become a very significant part of my life too.

I was naïve in a few other ways as well. The day Andrea casually mentioned and downplayed her bulimic habit to me was the day I was fooled into thinking that she could just stop throwing up whenever she wanted. She said it was just a "shortcut" that she used to stay slim when she didn't have time to exercise or when she felt sick to her stomach because she had overeaten. I also recalled that eating disorders were popular with fashion models and some of the stars in the entertainment industry ... so how bad could it be?

Secondly, I was totally unaware of the frequency of her binges and purges. Little did I know that she was binging and purging all day long, every day of the week. Once my eyes were opened to the extremity of the problem, I realized that her habit was a mental health disease and a very dangerous illness that required more support and intervention than I could ever provide on my own.

Finally, I thought if Andrea knew how strongly I disapproved of her habit then she might "smarten up" and just stop. So I got mad, and I got frustrated with her. Surprise, that didn't work either. Her refusal or inability to "stop for me" was one of the toughest and most humbling reality checks ... and for a number of years I wondered if my wife really loved me, and sometimes I resented her for that.

At the time, it felt like she needed her eating disorder more than she needed me. It often felt like she was "cheating on me", not with another man, but with food. There were lies, there was deceit. I even began "spying" on her. I would pretend to leave the house and then peek in the dining room window to see if she was pulling food out of the fridge or pantry to binge ... I couldn't believe that our relationship had gotten to that point, but that is the honest, ugly truth. So yes, there was mistrust and suspicion.

There was also a significant financial waste due to the cost of the food she binged and purged on. There was some arguing about that too. And, of course, there were many, many tears. I didn't believe her when she said that she still loved me. I would think, "How can she love me if she won't even do this for me?" I really didn't believe her when she said that she was trying to stop. At times, I wasn't even sure if "this was the person" that I had fallen for just a couple years ago. Again, I was simply frustrated and often mad. It took me several years to figure out that "quitting bulimia" is not just as easy as making a single, mind-over-matter decision. Later, I was told that an eating disorder can be ten times more difficult to quit than smoking. I'm not certain if that statistic is true, but I do know from the experience of being married to a woman that was both a bulimic and a smoker that an eating disorder was at least ten times more destructive and straining on our marriage than smoking. (Yes, Andrea is a "moderate" smoker. I would never downplay the harmful effects of smoking, but it is nowhere near as "damaging to our relationship" as bulimia was. I would be lying if I said I didn't want her to quit smoking too, but one thing at a time I suppose.)

As I look back on "our struggle" with bulimia, I wonder if some people are born with a more addictive personality than others. Is it possible that some people are "wired" a little differently, which makes them more prone to falling prey to an addiction? I don't know this for sure, but based on our experiences together I did wonder if Andrea was more susceptible to an illness such as an eating disorder or alcoholism … in comparison to someone like me? Was this just how she was built? I'm not even suggesting highly addictive substances like crystal meth, pain killers, or other prescription drugs, but instead more society-accepted items like fast-food, junk food and desserts, tobacco products, alcohol, and marijuana or activities such as exercise and gambling. Either way, whether she was "more susceptible or not", the fear of Andrea finding a replacement addiction to bulimia concerned me. Now that she had her "food addiction" under control, we needed to be mindful that bulimia was not replaced by another disordered "crutch". So, not that alcohol has ever taken over her life, nor do we consider it a serious concern at this time, but we are both quite cognisant that alcoholism could become the new coping mechanism. Due to concerns such as this, it is important to have ongoing communication to maintain or build a trusting and healthy relationship. Through our discussions, Andrea and I have concluded that we need to monitor all overindulgences, as any substance or action that is used to "forget" or temporarily numb emotions can become an addiction. It is also essential that the underlying mental health issues are not ignored after overcoming an addiction. Otherwise, a recovering addict could potentially fall back into a similar destructive cycle without much warning.

I have also learned that it takes a significant amount of time and reflection to feel emotionally and physically healthier. You have to stop beating yourself up over things from the past, as these thoughts are very damaging to self-worth. You have to prevent the "old negative tapes" from playing over and over again in your head, and replace them with new and more positive self-talk. To assist in this shift, participate in "daily check-ins" with your partner and family members. These "check-ins" can be a powerful tool if used routinely. These chats are honest, in the moment, conversations that will help dismiss negative self-talk and replace it with positive affirmations of the good in you. Realistically, the addiction will not disappear by chance and you cannot wish it away ... it will take hard work. You will feel frustrated when the healing process slows, or even regresses, and you will undoubtedly shed many tears along the way. Eventually, as I witnessed with Andrea, the destructive behaviour will slowly evolve and morph into healthier habits. It may sneak up on you, but you will know that you are healing once the negative self-talk lessens. You will slowly, but surely, begin to believe that you are a good person ... and that you deserve a better, happier, and healthier life.

As you can probably assume, this disordered eating journey was difficult on our relationship. There were many, many moments that tested our resolve and our commitment to each other within the first five years of our marriage. However, not all was bad. There were also many wonderful moments of happiness. The birth of our two boys was no doubt the highlight, along with many laughs and adventures with each other and our good friends. So did I ever, as Andrea often asked in the past, think of calling it quits or "packing it in"? I would be lying if I said it never crossed my mind. At times, I thought this can't be what a happy marriage should feel like. Maybe that was a self-centered thought or maybe it was a natural thought … I don't know, it just was. Our life together, at times, seemed a long way from happily-ever-after that is for sure.

I believe these feelings of marital doubt were not only because of what I was experiencing myself, but also out of concern for our home environment. I did not want to raise children in an environment that was filled with stress and dysfunction. Thankfully, by the time our boys were born, Andrea had made significant progress with her eating disorder and our boys were much too young still to comprehend the toxicity of their mother's mental health issues. So instead of flight, I chose fight. With some professional help, we fought this severe mental disorder together. I'm so glad we did, because Andrea gradually realized that she no longer needed the behavioural crutch of bulimia in her life, and she stopped binging and purging.

You are probably wondering if everything, including our marriage, is now "perfect". No, I don't think we can say that yet. Some of the scars of the past are still mending, but each day our trust in each other continues to grow. Maybe this writing process will help complete, or further facilitate, that healing. So, do I still have trust issues? Sometimes, but mostly just because I worry about Andrea's ongoing physical and mental health.

I also now recognize that not all of my negative feelings about our relationship were strictly due to Andrea's eating disorder. I have "stuff" or emotional baggage from my childhood too, which undoubtedly act as emotional *triggers* for me today. I don't think I would have admitted that prior to this project. Andrea has truly inspired me with her bravery to be open and honest about her darkest and ugliest secrets. Secrets that she now shares only in the hopes of possibly helping a young girl, boy, adolescent, or adult climb out of their dark hole of emotional struggles. Because of her bravery, I too am slowly learning to become more open with her about my own dysfunctional childhood.

So here is a bit of my story … My parents' marriage and the home environment that my siblings and I grew up in was horrible. I don't know how else to say it. There was verbal and physical abuse, there was alcoholism, there was depression, and there was even an attempt of suicide through a prescription drug overdose. No kids should have to see the things that we saw and experienced. Sadly though, many children in this world do experience what we did, and much worse. Society doesn't have to look too far when wondering why there seem to be more and more mental health issues in children. I believe one of the keys to well-adjusted and mentally-healthy children begins with nurturing parents that set healthy limits for their children.

I can honestly say that it wasn't until my parents' "golden years" that I learned to forgive them, love them again, and finally feel at peace with them. The biggest improvement was when my dad stopped abusing alcohol. Ever since I can remember, alcohol was the deep-seated evil in our home, my parents' relationship, and in our childhood. For a man who was well-respected in most public circles and who cared very much for his children when sober, our dad transformed into a mean-spirited and abusive caregiver when intoxicated. My mother was a victim of his verbal and physical abuse, yet I often wondered why she didn't just get out of the marriage. Not only to protect herself, but also her children from the dysfunction of alcoholism ... or at least, force my dad to get the help that he needed for his illness. I also now under-stand that my mother suffered from depression at that time, possibly triggered by the abusive experiences inflicted upon her. Because of her lack of education and ability to support us, I assume that she resigned herself to a "survival mode" in order to keep the family together. I'm sure she thought, and hoped, that things would eventually get better. I feel like her gamble came at a big price, because the dysfunction lasted for many years. It robbed all of my siblings and myself from a "normal and happy" childhood, specifically when we were behind the private and closed doors of our small-town home.

For the most part, my dad quit drinking alcohol around the same time the boys came into our life. I'm glad he did, as my kids got to know a more caring grandpa instead of the Dad I grew up resenting during my childhood. I certainly cannot speak for my siblings, as they had their very own personalized experiences as kids, but it is beyond me how I came out the other side of my childhood without more emotional scars. Maybe someone above was looking out for me. Today, my biggest goal in life is to provide my children with an emotionally stable and loving home. Not that we spoil our kids, far from it actually. We definitely teach them right from wrong and at the same time we want them to have fond memories of their childhood. I realize the most precious gift we can give our children is time spent together. At times, considering my childhood and Andrea's mental health struggles, I think it would have been quite easy for our family to fall into a cycle of dysfunction. Thankfully, we were able to find a different path and create a very caring and loving home environment for our boys. In the end, we all have choices to make and promises to keep to ourselves. Sometimes, that is just a little harder to do when it means changing who we are today in order to become someone better, or healthier, tomorrow.

Andrea is a wonderful mother and I know she would do just about anything for Ajay and Sammy. Maybe that is where some of her amazing strength came from in this grueling fight. If I learned anything from those early turmoil-filled years of our marriage that I can pass along to those in a relationship where someone suffers from an addiction, like an eating disorder ... Please, please, try not to take things too personally. This process won't be easy. You will feel moments of tremendous disappointment. You will most certainly need to remember that your partner has a behavioural addiction and a mental illness, so that you do not take their deceit personally. They will lie to you, and they will do things that will make you mistrust them ... and they will make you feel insignificant. Not purposely, but because they are ill.

If you truly care about them, then I hope you are able to find a way to separate the disease from the person. If you are able to do that, then I am confident that you will discover that they do still love you, that they do not want to hurt you, nor do they want to make you feel insignificant. What they need from you is your unconditional love and your patience as they try to survive the struggles inside their head. You will have to find the right balance between "supporting them, without enabling them". In our case, the delicate process of trying to establish open, honest, critical, but yet trusting conversation took several years to develop before it transformed into dialogue that was positive, meaningful, and relationship-strengthening. That being said, it is unfair to believe that "you can fix them" alone. However, with the support of professional counsellors, you can assist in their healing journey. Ultimately though, the partner, the child, the friend or the family member that is struggling with the eating disorder must do the "heavy work" themselves, in order to reincarnate a healthier and more respectful self-image.

Also remember that this disordered eating behaviour did not take a hold of your loved-one overnight, so realistically it will be a very lengthy and difficult struggle to overcome its grasp as well. However, I truly believe that once you come to terms with the turmoil that is created within this vicious cycle of addiction, and once you better understand the continuum of healing that a disordered-eater must travel, you will then have the strength and the understanding to stand beside them throughout this very emotional fight for mental wellness and happiness.

Respectfully, Mick Parmar

A FINAL THANK YOU

There are so many people that I need to recognize with a Thank You. I would like to start with the *BridgePoint Center For Eating Disorders* in Milden, Saskatchewan. I truly don't know which direction my life would have taken if I hadn't found out about this life-changing facility. I admire the personal and non-judgemental approach they take in counselling their disordered eating participants. The environment that the staff has created not only made me feel safe and secure, but it assured me that I was not alone in this battle. Their therapy processes helped me peel through the many layers of my mental illness so that I could feel "whole and present" once again. After feeling "Alone in a Crowd" for so many years, I finally felt a glimmer of hope and healing because this program. I sincerely thank all of the staff and the participants for giving me the tools, the insight, and the strength to eliminate bulimic habits from my life. The need for more disordered eating facilities such as BridgePoint cannot be overstated ... without a doubt these facilities not only change lives, but they also save them.

I am also blessed to have many wonderful friends and family members in my life. Let me start with my friend Debbie. We have such a strong and unique bond because of all that we went through together at BridgePoint. I can't say enough about how she helped me heal. The bond we made there was life-changing ... call it fate, call it chance, call it what you want, but when Debbie and I connected at BridgePoint we developed a relationship that made us both better people. To this day, we continue to support each other and are good friends. When nobody else could understand my disordered eating struggles, Debbie would "get me". No matter how many months may go by without chatting, whenever one of us makes a phone call to the other, we seem to just pick up where we left off.

Next I would like to thank my best-friend-forever, Christine. I am truly blessed to have her in my life. I can't even count the times that she has "rescued me". Our unconditional friendship is very special to me. Another incredible lady is my friend Tracey, who has been there for me in so many caring ways. A special thank you to Julie as well, for lending an ear when needed. I sincerely appreciate all of these beautiful women and their families for being such good friends to me and my family.

Now to my immediate family. We are a tight knit bunch and my siblings have always been there for me. It was heartwarming when Tammy and Geoff came along, with my parents, to the Family and Friends weekend at BridgePoint. I realized the true meaning of family then. I also know that my special sis Kim would have been there too if she was able. She has always been a reliable support in my not-so-good days. The fact that my whole family was willing to participate in my recovery was inspiring. I still have all the inspirational cards that Tammy and Kim sent to me over the years. I am so lucky to have the siblings that I do.

I have a hard time putting into words the way I feel about my parents. My mom is the rock, slightly cracked from overuse maybe, that holds us all together. She would do just about anything for her kids. She has a heart of gold, and in my opinion, is the greatest Mom and Grandmother in the world. I hope I can be as good of a mother for my kids as she has been to me. As for my dad, I wondered if he would begin charging me rent considering all the nights I needed to spend at their house over the years. Dad, your unconditional love means the world to me. You too are the greatest Dad and Papa that God ever made.

Finally to my beloved boys, Ajay and Sammy. No matter what the future holds always know that Mom and Dad love you more than anything in the world. We are very proud of the beautiful and caring boys you are now and the amazing young men that you will undoubtedly become someday. Thank you for not giving up on Mom.

With love, Andrea

THE BUTTERFLY

*once tattered and injured,
there seemed to be no hope
nor any end to the despair,
then one morning something happened
a heavy weight lifted away,
so with the support of others
and so much difficult work on my own,
I learned to forgive and respect myself*

*so now just like the Butterfly,
i have risen from my cocoon
still a bit fragile and uncertain,
yet present and no longer afraid
i'm ready to fly high and explore,
wherever these winds will take me
to spread healing and hope,
and live a life reborn*

**Learn to forgive, respect, and love yourself
and you will heal too.**

Andrea and Mick Parmar

ABOUT THE AUTHOR

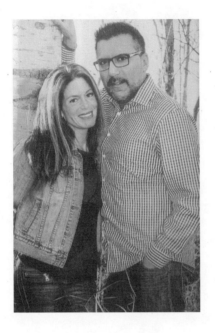

Andrea (Gilbert) Parmar grew up in Regina, Saskatchewan, Canada. She moved to Langenburg in 2000, where she now resides with her husband Mick and their two boys Ajay and Sammy. Andrea has worked as a Registered Psychiatric Nurse (RPN) since 1994 until her recent diagnosis of Multiple Sclerosis. She passionately strives to increase public awareness regarding the complex issues of disordered eating. Andrea hopes that by sharing her story of recovery from a "secret battle" with self-harm, anxiety, depression and bulimia that she will not only instill hope in those that suffer from a mental illness, but also act as an advocate for the funding of in-patient eating disorder facilities and early intervention programs in schools.

Printed in Canada